Management of Multi-Drug Resistant TB Treatment: Social Work Perspective

Management of Multi-Drug Resistant TB Treatment: Social Work Perspective

Authors

Dr. Murugesan Periyasamy

Dr. Sathyamurthi Karibeeran

ALLIED PUBLISHERS PVT. LTD.

Noida • Mumbai • Kolkata • Chennai • Bangalore

ALLIED PUBLISHERS PRIVATE LIMITED

D-5, Sector-2, **Noida**–201 301
Ph. Nos.: 0120-4320295/2542557/4352866 • E-mail: delhi.books@alliedpublishers.com

17 Chittaranjan Avenue, **Kolkata**–700072
Ph.: 033-22129618 • E-mail: cal.books@alliedpublishers.com

15 J.N. Heredia Marg, Ballard Estate, **Mumbai**–400001
Ph.: 022-42126969 • E-mail: mumbai.books@alliedpublishers.com

No. 25/10, Commander-in-Chief Road, Ethiraj Lane (Next to Post Office)
Egmore, **Chennai**–600008
Ph.: 044-28223938 • E-mail: chennai.books@alliedpublishers.com

P.B. No. 9932, No. 15, 3rd Floor (Next to Vijaya Bank), 5th Cross, Gandhinagar,
Karnataka, **Bangalore**–560009, Ph.: 080-41530285 / 22386239
E-mail: bngl.books@alliedpublishers.com

Website: www.alliedpublishers.com

ISBN: 978-93-89934-78-6

Published by Sunil Sachdev and printed by Ravi Sachdev at Allied Publishers Pvt. Ltd., D-5, Sector-2, Noida–201 301

Preface

On World Tuberculosis Day (Sunday, March 24), the National Institute of Allergy and Infectious Diseases (NIAID), a division of the National Institutes of Health, joins our partners in reaffirming our commitment to ending the tuberculosis (TB) pandemic and remembering those who have died as a result of the disease. This year's commemoration will include the 2023 theme "Yes! We Can End TB!" as a recognition to the strong momentum of the TB response in many high-burden countries, aided by the dedication of TB stakeholders throughout the world. On this day, NIAID recognizes the leadership of persons impacted by tuberculosis, their communities, and civil society.

Tuberculosis is a disease caused by Mycobacterium tuberculosis. As many as two billion people worldwide have latent M. tuberculosis infections, which have a 5 10% probability of progressing to active illness over the course of their lives. The World Health Organization predicts that 10.6 million people will have active tuberculosis by 2022, with 1.3 million being children and 1.3 million dying from the disease. The Centers for Disease Control and Prevention estimate that up to 13 million people in the United States have latent M. tuberculosis, and that 8,331 people will develop active TB in 2022, representing a 5.9% increase over 2021 numbers and the second consecutive year of rising TB incidence. There were 602 TB-related deaths in the United States in 2021.

MDR-TB, commonly known as drug-resistant tuberculosis, is a major threat to global public health, particularly in low- and middle-income countries. Most of the development of MDR-TB is attributable to ineffective clinical outcomes and suboptimal regimen adherence. Approximately 50% of MDR-TB patients fail to complete treatment (WHO). Prolonged treatment length (usually 24 months or longer) and drug toxicity contribute to treatment adherence problems and result in such poor outcomes. A prolonged and thorough treatment plan includes powerful medications that can result in a variety of mental health issues, including psychosis. It has a higher rate of follow-up loss and worse cure outcomes than drug-sensitive tuberculosis, as well as a higher case fatality rate (TB). Other components of psychological ill-health, which are not often addressed, are left to fester and grow. Globally, fewer than half of MDR-TB patients complete their treatment. A significant major reason for these poor outcomes is the lengthy treatment period (which is generally 24 months or longer) and drug toxicity, which results in poor adherence to treatment. Psychological issues are also known to aggravate MDR-TB in some cases.

People with multidrug-resistant tuberculosis (MDR-TB) have difficulty finding effective treatment alternatives, as there are just a few treatments, they have to continue treatment for a long time, and the treatments themselves are toxic. Despite advancements in microbiological and clinical research into MDR-TB, psychosocial aspects of the illness are limited and poorly understood. The aim of this book is to explain the MDR-TB patients' treatment experiences, family support, institutional support, physiological distress, stigma and discrimination, and overall health to understand their perspective. The specific objectives are to assess the socio-economic profile of MDR-TB patients, their general health status of MDR-TB patients, and their psychosocial well-being of MDR-TB patients. The book also aimed to understand the understand the stigma & discrimination of MDR-TB patient and to understand the understand the support system for MDR-TB patients.

This book designed at describing the background characteristic of persons affected by Multi Drug-Resistant TB and their psych-social well-being, socio-economic condition, general health status, psychological distress and self-stigma. The researcher adopted the descriptive research design to explain these background characteristics and explain its relationships with other variables. The TB treatment profiles collected included the duration of TB illness, patient previous treatment, from where previous treatment was taken, money spent on private treatment etc. The family support profile included the details of family support during this illness, isolation by the family members, sleeping pattern, taking food with family members and usage of separate glass and plate. The institutional support profile includes distance to the government hospital, opinion on government hospital treatment, opinion on government hospital staff service and sources of taking daily DOT's. Besides, the research book examines the psychosocial well-being of MDR tuberculosis patients in Chennai Corporation. As a result, the research study focuses on describing the psychosocial characteristics of MDR-TB patients, which serves as a descriptive research design. The total number of patients on the list was 323 and of the researcher removed seven deceased patients, another nineteen who lost to follow up (LFU). Hence the 26 patients were not considered for this book. And finally, two hundred and ninety (297) were eligible for the book. Hence 297 is considered for the sample of the study.

An informed consent form was given to two hundred and ninety-seven (297) MDR-TB patients and requested them to participate in the book. Those who are willing to provide the written informed consent process were completed. Then the interview was conducted in the health facility (TU) itself as per the patient's convenient time. Eight patients were not willing to participate in the book due to their personal and privacy issues. A total of 289 respondents who were willing to participate in the book were enrolled and interviewed. The data has collected from two hundred and eighty-nine (289) MDR-TB patients from 5 Health Districts in Chennai (North, East, West, South and Central) of Chennai Corporation, those who are diagnosed for MDR-TB and taking treatment under the National Tuberculosis Elimination programme (NTEP) formerly known as the Revised National Tuberculosis Programme (RNTCP).

Of the total 289 MDR-TB patients, the total number of male MDR-TB patients was 72.7 per cent. Among the male MDR-TB patients, in North Chennai (24.6%), East Chennai (19.7%), Central Chennai (13.8%), West Chennai (7.6%) and South Chennai (6.9%). Female respondents made up approximately 27.3 per cent of the total, with respondents from North Chennai (6.2%), East Chennai (6.9%), Central Chennai (6.6%), West Chennai (4.8%), and South Chennai (2.8%). The majority of the respondents (61.6%) stated that they were isolated by their family members as a result of their MDR-TB. Some respondents (38.4%) claimed that they were not isolated by their family members. It was reported that more than half (53.3%) of the MDR-TB patients reported that the nearest government health facility was more than 5 kilometres away from their residence. Of the total number of responders, 46.7% stated that the nearest government health facility or government hospital is less than 5 kilometres away.

It was revealed that more than half (58.1%) of the MDR-TB patients reported that the behaviour of government health workers and the quality of their treatment at the government health facility were satisfactory. Patients who were satisfied with the behaviour of government health workers and the quality of their treatment accounted for 41.9% of the total. More than half (58.1) MDR-TB patients reported that the behaviour and service of government staff were good in public health. 41.9% of patients had positive behaviour and good service in their discussions with health care personnel. 72.7 per cent (10.4) of those who were male had a low environmental mastery level. However, there was a moderate self-acceptance level (46.7) per cent of the patients and a high level of environmental mastery for 10.4 per cent of the patients. The majority (72.7 per cent) of respondents were male, and there was evidence of a moderate level of a good relationship, with almost half (46.4 per cent) of respondents having a favourable relationship.

The majority of respondents, 72.7 per cent, were male, and there was evidence of a moderate level of purpose in life, with almost half (45.7%) of respondents indicating a moderate level of life purpose. It is noticed that patients aged 18 to 30 years had a moderate level of self-acceptance (24.6%) and 14.5% of them had a moderate level of self-acceptance, while patients aged 51 to 60 years had a moderate level of self-acceptance (25.3%) and 13.8% of them had a moderate level of self-acceptance. The majority of respondents (72.7 per cent) were male, and there was evidence of a moderate level of psychological well-being, with almost half (40.5%) reporting a sense of well-being. When compared to females, 27.3 per cent of them exhibit signs of moderate psychological well-being (17.3 per cent). The book found that the age and education level of the MDR-TB patients were associated with the presence of a strong family support system. With regard to family support, there was no correlation between age and education in the MDR-TB patients. The association between the monthly income of MDR tuberculosis patients and the level of family assistance was found to be related.

It was found that MDR-TB patients who have taken previous therapy for TB are strongly connected to their family support. In addition, it was discovered that the duration of TB disease of MDR-TB patients was significantly linked to the level of family assistance provided to them. There is a considerable relationship between the cost of private TB treatment and the amount of family support provided to the MDR-TB patient. This means that it has also been found that there is no connection between the duration of the TB problem and the level of family support for patients who have extensively drug-resistant TB. It has been found that the well-being of MDR-TB patients diagnosed with multidrug-resistant tuberculosis (MDR-TB) varies depending on age, gender, ethnicity, religion, social standing, personal attributes, and socioeconomic status. Poverty and illiteracy, when combined with several other factors, have an impact on a person's overall health, psychological well-being, and sense of personal shame. To achieve this there are many ways such as imparting basic education to all, providing employment opportunities, improving the health facilities, creating good health infrastructure facilities and involving various other stakeholders. Promotion of health facilities for the dreaded disease like TB and MDR-TB also would go a long way in addressing their health problems.

This book could be very helpful for future social workers and other researchers who wish to perform further research on this topic, as it aims to improve MDR-TB patients' psychological well-being. To build on these preliminary findings and provide information on established psychosocial interventions that could be replicated in TB control programmes, large-scale multicentre investigations and randomised control trials are strongly recommended.

The primary goal of this book is to assist individuals who are not experts in drug-resistant tuberculosis but must comprehend and assist in advising and managing such cases in ordinary practice. It offers an overview of the most recent diagnostic tests and treatment regimens for various kinds of drug-resistant TB. In this book, we have included both quantitative and qualitative research on patients "in the real world". I genuinely hope that this initiative achieves its goals.

Acknowledgement

I'm extremely grateful to Dr. K. Sathyamurthi, PhD, my Research Supervisor, who played a decisive role throughout my PhD work with his relentless support, valuable advice, constructive criticism, practical suggestions, ingenious guidance, persistent motivation and profound belief in my work. I would like to extend my deepest gratitude to Dr. S. Raja Samuel, Principal, School of Social Work, for his support, and suggestions. Dr. Enoch Arokiasamy, Assistant Professor for his motivation and support. I am grateful to the University of Madras and the Madras School of Social Work in Chennai for providing me with the opportunity to pursue a doctoral degree.

My heartfelt thanks go to Dr. Mahalingam Kannan, former principal, and Captain Dr. D.V.P. Raja, founder of Madurai Institute of Social Sciences, who have supported me to complete my studies. Dr. O. Muthiah, Head of Folklore & Performing Arts and Modern Literature; Dr. M. William Baskaran, Professor & Head of Peace Studies, Gandhian Thought, Conflict Resolution, Transformation Shanti Sena, and Counseling; and Dean Dr. G. Palani Durai, Department of Politics and Public Administration; Professor Boraiyan, Department of Extension Education, Gandhigram Deemed University.

I'd want to express my thanks to the Madras School of Social Work academics, as well as the office staff, library staff, IT support staff, and all other teaching and non-teaching personnel of Madras School of Social Work in Chennai.

Dr. Soumya Swaminathan, former Director-General of ICMR and Health Secretary of the Department of Health Research, Ministry of Health and Family Welfare, New Delhi, is currently working as a Chief Scientist for the World Health Organization (WHO). Dr. Raman R. Gangakhedkar is the Director of the Division of Epidemiology and Communicable Diseases (ECD) of the Indian Council of Medical Research in New Delhi. Dr. Sanjay Mehendale, Dr. Srikanth Tripathy, former Director In-Charge, and Dr. Padma

Priyadharsini, Director of ICMR-National Institute for Research in Tuberculosis for their approval and support to Pursue my PhD.

I would like to express my sincere thanks to the Commissioner and Deputy Director (Health) and Dr. Jegadheesan. The City Health Officer, Greater Chennai Corporation, permitted me to conduct a study at the Chennai Corporation Tuberculosis Unit attached to the Urban Primary health centre, Chennai. Dr. Lavanya, District Tuberculosis Officer, Chennai and the whole staff of the DTO office, Pulianthop, Chennai for the list of TB patients and necessary data. My special thanks to Medical Officer–TB Control (MO-TC), Senior Treatment Supervisor (STS) and Senior Tuberculosis Laboratory Supervisor (STLS), Health Visitor (HV), DR TB Co-Ordinators, Lab Technicians and other Administration staff etc.

I acknowledge the study participants (MDR-TB patients) for their willingness to participate in the study and the time spent on the quantitative and qualitative interviews. A special thanks to all the respondents' family members who participated in the In-depth Interview.

Dr. Beena. E. Thomas, former Head of the Department of Social and Behavioural Research (DSBR), ICMR-NIRT, Mrs Sudha Ganapathy, Mrs, Geetha Ramani Shunmugam, Mrs Mohana Rani Suhadev, Mrs Meenalochini Dileep, Mrs Shella Fredric's, Mrs K. Jagannatharao, Mrs Niruparani Charless, Mr Raja Sakthivel, Mr Thiruvalluvan, Mrs Chandra Suresh, Mrs Kalaiselvi, Mrs Deepalakshmi, Dr. Stephen and Dr. Karikalan, Head of the Department of Social and Behavioural Research (DSBR), ICMR-NIRT, Chennai, deserve special thanks for all of their advice and guidance throughout my PhD journey.

The completion of my PhD research work and thesis writing would not have been possible if not for the unparalleled support, extensive care, constant nurturing, and boundless tolerance of my beloved wife, Mrs Muthamil Sheela Murugesan, District Protection Officer, Department of Social Welfare, Collector office, Villupuram, and my dear parents, Mr Periyasamy (Late), Mrs Seerangammal, and P. Ponnammal, to whom I'm deeply grateful. I cannot begin to express my appreciation to my treasured offspring, Mr P.M. Buvanesh and P.M Rokesh, who, despite their want of my time and attention, are attuned to my busy work schedules.

Mr P. Manivel, Mrs Eswari, P.M. Boopesh, P. Krishnamoorthy, Mrs Ambiga, Mrs Periyakkal, Mr Rajasekar, R. Prakash, R.Naveen, P. Ramathilagam, Master. V. Aravindh, Mr P. Ganesan, Mr John Vetrivel, Pramila John, Ms Hanukka, and Harshit, for their continuous encouragement. Mr M. Chinnapa, Mrs P. Marthal, Dr. P. Susilal, MBBS., Retired Ophthalmologist, Government Medical College Hospital, Asaripallam, Nagercoil, as well as my in-laws Mr Jegatheesh, Mr Sujey, Mrs Radhika, Mrs Beaulina Wilson, and all other relatives for bearing with the nature of my profession.

Mr Nawaj Shaikh, PhD Scholar, ICMR-NARI, Pune, Mr Rony Moral, and Jacob Prem Kumar, ICMR-NIRT, Chennai, are acknowledged for their support. Dr. J. Vignesh Kumar, Social Scientist, Christian Medical College & Hospital, Vellore, Mrs R. Kalaivani, Treasurer, Thambiraan Foundation, Dindigul and Dr. Babu Thiyagarajan, Consultant, Madurai are all grateful for their assistance.

I'm also appreciative of the technical assistance provided by all of the personnel at Excel Copying Centre in Chennai, particularly Mr. Shunmugasundaram. I'd want to express my appreciation to everyone who assisted me in any manner during my education. I can't go without acknowledging the heavenly blessings that have been showered upon me for all of my achievements.

Dr. P. Murugesan, ***PhD***

List of Abbreviations

DR-TB	Drug-resistant tuberculosis
DR-TBC	Drug-Resistant Tuberculosis Centre
HF	Health facility
Hr-TB	Isoniazid-resistant TB
IP	Intensive phase
LFU	Loss to follow up
MDR-TB	Multi-drug resistant TB
MO	Medical Officer
NIRT	National Institute for Research in Tuberculosis
NPY	Nikshay Poshan Yojana
NSP	National strategic plan
NTEP	National Tuberculosis Elimination Programme
PMDT	Programmatic management of drug-resistant tuberculosis
PT	Previously treated
R	Rifampicin
RNTCP	Revised National Tuberculosis Control Programme
RR-TB	Rifampicin resistant tuberculosis
S	Streptomycin
SDG	Sustainable Development Goals
SLD	Second-line anti-TB drugs
SLI	Second-line injectable
TB	Tuberculosis
TBI	Tuberculosis infection

TU	TB unit
WHO	World Health Organization
XDR-TB	Extensively-drug resistant TB

Contents

Abstract

Introduction

MDR-TB, commonly known as drug-resistant tuberculosis, is a major threat to global public health, particularly in low- and middle-income countries. Most of the development of MDR-TB is attributable to ineffective clinical outcomes and suboptimal regimen adherence. Approximately 50% of MDR-TB patients fail to complete treatment (WHO). Prolonged treatment length (usually 24 months or longer) and drug toxicity contribute to treatment adherence problems and result in such poor outcomes. A prolonged and thorough treatment plan includes powerful medications that can result in a variety of mental health issues, including psychosis. It has a higher rate of follow-up loss and worse cure outcomes than drug-sensitive tuberculosis, as well as a higher case fatality rate (TB). Other components of psychological ill-health, which are not often addressed, are left to fester and grow. Globally, fewer than half of MDR-TB patients complete their treatment. A significant major reason for these poor outcomes is the lengthy treatment period (which is generally 24 months or longer) and drug toxicity, which results in poor adherence to treatment. Psychological issues are also known to aggravate MDR-TB in some cases. People with multidrug-resistant tuberculosis (MDR-TB) have difficulty finding effective treatment alternatives, as there are just a few treatments, they have to continue treatment for a long time, and the treatments themselves are toxic. Despite advancements in microbiological and clinical research into MDR-TB, psychosocial aspects of the illness are limited and poorly understood.

Aim: The aim of this book is to study MDR-TB patients' treatment experiences, family support, institutional support, physiological distress, stigma and discrimination, and overall health to understand their perspective. The specific objectives are to assess the socio-economic profile of MDR-TB patients, their general health status of MDR-TB patients, their psychosocial well-being of MDR-TB patients. The book also aimed to understand the understand the stigma &

discrimination of MDR-TB patient and to understand the understand the support system for MDR-TB patients.

Methods: The study utilised a descriptive research study design. The research study aimed at describing the background characteristic of persons affected by Multi Drug-Resistant TB and their psych-social well-being, socio-economic condition, general health status, psychological distress and self-stigma. The authors adopted the descriptive research design to explain these background characteristics and explain its relationships with other variables. The TB treatment profiles collected included the duration of TB illness, patient previous treatment, from where previous treatment was taken, money spent on private treatment etc. The family support profile included the details of family support during this illness, isolation by the family members, sleeping pattern, taking food with family members and usage of separate glass and plate. The institutional support profile includes distance to the government hospital, opinion on government hospital treatment, opinion on government hospital staff service and sources of taking daily DOT's. Besides, the research study focuses the psychosocial well-being of MDR tuberculosis patients in Chennai Corporation. As a result, the research book focuses on describing the psychosocial characteristics of MDR-TB patients, which serves as a descriptive research design. The total number of patients on the list was 323 and of the authors removed seven deceased patients, another nineteen who lost to follow up (LFU). Hence the 26 patients were not considered for this study. And finally, two hundred and ninety (297) were eligible for the study. Hence 297 is considered for the sample of the study.

An informed consent form was given to two hundred and ninety-seven (297) MDR-TB patients and requested them to participate in the study. Those who are willing to provide the written informed consent process were completed. Then the interview was conducted in the health facility (TU) itself as per the patient's convenient time. Eight patients were not willing to participate in the book due to their personal and privacy issues. A total of 289 respondents who were willing to participate in the study were enrolled and interviewed. The data has collected from two hundred and eighty-nine (289) MDR-TB patients from 5 Health Districts in Chennai (North, East, West,

South and Central) of Chennai Corporation, those who are diagnosed for MDR-TB and taking treatment under the National Tuberculosis Elimination programme (NTEP) formerly known as the Revised National Tuberculosis Programme (RNTCP).

Results: Of the total 289 MDR-TB patients, the total number of male MDR-TB patients was 72.7 per cent. Among the male MDR-TB patients, in North Chennai (24.6%), East Chennai (19.7%), Central Chennai (13.8%), West Chennai (7.6%) and South Chennai (6.9%). Female respondents made up approximately 27.3 per cent of the total, with respondents from North Chennai (6.2%), East Chennai (6.9%), Central Chennai (6.6%), West Chennai (4.8%), and South Chennai (2.8%).

The majority of the respondents (61.6%) stated that they were isolated by their family members as a result of their MDR-TB. Some respondents (38.4%) claimed that they were not isolated by their family members. It was reported that more than half (53.3%) of the MDR-TB patients reported that the nearest government health facility was more than 5 kilometres away from their residence. Of the total number of responders, 46.7% stated that the nearest government health facility or government hospital is less than 5 kilometres away.

It was revealed that more than half (58.1%) of the MDR-TB patients reported that the behaviour of government health workers and the quality of their treatment at the government health facility were satisfactory. Patients who were satisfied with the behaviour of government health workers and the quality of their treatment accounted for 41.9% of the total.

More than half (58.1) MDR-TB patients reported that the behaviour and service of government staff were good in public health. 41.9% of patients had positive behaviour and good service in their discussions with health care personnel. 72.7 per cent (10.4) of those who were male had a low environmental mastery level. However, there was a moderate self-acceptance level (46.7) per cent of the patients and a high level of environmental mastery for 10.4 per cent of the patients. The majority (72.7 per cent) of respondents were male, and there was evidence of a moderate level of a good relationship, with almost half (46.4 per cent) of respondents having a favourable relationship.

The majority of respondents, 72.7 per cent, were male, and there was evidence of a moderate level of purpose in life, with almost half (45.7%) of respondents indicating a moderate level of life purpose. It is noticed that patients aged 18 to 30 years had a moderate level of self-acceptance (24.6%) and 14.5% of them had a moderate level of self-acceptance, while patients aged 51 to 60 years had a moderate level of self-acceptance (25.3%) and 13.8% of them had a moderate level of self-acceptance. The majority of respondents (72.7 per cent) were male, and there was evidence of a moderate level of psychological well-being, with almost half (40.5%) reporting a sense of well-being. When compared to females, 27.3 per cent of them exhibit signs of moderate psychological well-being (17.3 per cent).

Discussion: The book found that the age and education level of the MDR-TB patients were associated with the presence of a strong family support system. With regard to family support, there was no correlation between age and education in the MDR-TB patients. The association between the monthly income of MDR tuberculosis patients and the level of family assistance was found to be related.

It was found that MDR-TB patients who have taken previous therapy for TB are strongly connected to their family support. In addition, it was discovered that the duration of TB disease of MDR-TB patients was significantly linked to the level of family assistance provided to them. There is a considerable relationship between the cost of private TB treatment and the amount of family support provided to the MDR-TB patient. This means that it has also been found that there is no connection between the duration of the TB problem and the level of family support for patients who have extensively drug-resistant TB.

Conclusion: It has been found that the well-being of MDR-TB patients diagnosed with multidrug-resistant tuberculosis (MDR-TB) varies depending on age, gender, ethnicity, religion, social standing, personal attributes, and socioeconomic status. Poverty and illiteracy, when combined with several other factors, have an impact on a person's overall health, psychological well-being, and sense of personal shame. To achieve this there are many ways such as imparting basic education to all, providing employment opportunities, improving the health facilities, creating good health infrastructure facilities and involving various other stakeholders. Promotion of health facilities for the dreaded disease like TB and MDR-TB also would go a long way in addressing their health problems.

This book could be very helpful for future social workers and other authors who wish to perform further research on this topic, as it aims to improve MDR-TB patients' psychological well-being. To build on these preliminary findings and provide information on established psychosocial interventions that could be replicated in TB control programmes, large-scale multicentre investigations and randomised control trials are strongly recommended.

CHAPTER 1

Materials

Tuberculosis (TB) is a contagious infection that spreads from person to person. Mycobacterium tuberculosis is the bacillus that causes TB. Tuberculosis spreads through the air when an infected person coughs, sneezes, or even speaks. People nearby may become infected if they are exposed to such droplets for an extended period. Individuals who have tuberculosis of the lungs are more prone to transfer the bacterium to people with whom they spend daily time, such as family members, acquaintances, and co-workers. When someone inhales tuberculosis germs, the bacteria colonise the lungs. Once the immune system of that individual is weakened, the germs begin to grow. Although the disease is most commonly associated with the lungs (pulmonary tuberculosis), it can also affect other organs such as the brain, kidneys, or spine (extrapulmonary TB). *(World Health Organisation-fact sheet, 2021).*

According to the World Health Organization (WHO), one-third of the world's population has latent tuberculosis (LTB), which implies that individuals have been infected with tuberculosis germs but are not yet unwell with the disease and so cannot spread the disease. 10% of persons infected with tuberculosis germs are at risk of developing tuberculosis over their lives. Individuals with weakened immune systems, such as those who have HIV, malnutrition, or diabetes, or those who use cigarettes. Tuberculosis (TB) is a highly contagious sickness that spreads through contact. Mycobacterium tuberculosis is the bacteria that cause tuberculosis. are at a -increased risk of contracting tuberculosis. While a person develops active tuberculosis disease, the symptoms (cough, fever, night sweats, and weight loss, for example) may stay moderate for months, which is one of the primary reasons for delaying treatment and resulting in the spread of the germs to others. When a person becomes infected with tuberculosis, they can infect up to 10–15 individuals who come into touch with the sick person over one year.

Additionally, it is believed that a considerable proportion of individuals afflicted with tuberculosis die without receiving adequate treatment. Since ancient times, humanity has been aware of tuberculosis. Historically, this disease was known by a variety of names, including consumption (owing to the patient's significant weight loss and the way the virus looked to "devour" the body), phthisis pulmonarias, and the white plague (due to the extreme pallor seen among those infected). Despite the advancement of sophisticated and scientific procedures for screening, diagnosis, and treatment, one-third of the world's population remains infected. In poor countries, approximately 90% of people are infected with TB. With the emergence of HIV infection, TB has had a dramatic resurgence, with more than 8 million new cases reported each year and over 2 million fatalities.

Global TB Burden

Tuberculosis is most prevalent in individuals during their prime years of productivity. However, individuals of all ages are in danger. Worldwide, an estimated 10.0 million (range, 8.9–11.0 million) persons contracted tuberculosis in 2019, including 5.6 million men, 3.2 million women, and 1.2 million children. HIV-positive individuals accounted for 8.2 per cent of the total. India, Indonesia, China, the Philippines, Pakistan, Nigeria, Bangladesh, and South Africa accounted for more than two-thirds of the world total. 1.4 million individuals will die of tuberculosis in 2019, including 208000 (177000–242000) persons living with HIV. Over 95% of the illnesses and fatalities occurred in poor nations. *(WHO Fact sheet 2020).*

TB Burden in India

India is classified as having a "high TB burden." Country. According to estimates, India contributes to more than 25% of the worldwide tuberculosis burden and the illness kills more than 400,000 individuals in the country each year. While the Indian government has been working toward eliminating tuberculosis in the nation by 2025, the COVID-19 epidemic last year threw a wrench in the works. The COVID-19 pandemic poses a danger to undo recent gains in lowering the burden of tuberculosis illness and increasing access to care. The epidemic has had a significant effect on tuberculosis health care. For the period January–June 2020, data from numerous high-TB burden nations suggest a dramatic decline in TB notifications. According to the WHO's assessment, a 50% decrease in tuberculosis case detection over three months may result in over 400,000 extra tuberculosis deaths in 2020 WHO has begun collaborating closely with partners and civil society to assist the nation in ensuring the continuation of key health care services, including those for tuberculosis. *(Global Tuberculosis Report 2020).*

Drug-Resistant (DR) Tuberculosis

Drug-resistant tuberculosis (DR TB) is a growing issue that complicates tuberculosis management. Rifampicin is a critical component of TB treatments. Resistance to this agent is frequently linked with resistance to isoniazid, culminating in multidrug-resistant tuberculosis (MDR-TB). Although evidence of single-drug resistance was discovered as early as 1948, strains of the illness were later shown to be resistant to two or even more medicines. The worst-case scenario for a patient with tuberculosis is when the illness develops resistance to two or more of the conventional medicines.

Drug resistance can be a tragedy not only for the patient but also for others, as the sick might spread drug-resistant germs to others (Sir John Crofton, 1959). Globally, 465,000 individuals were diagnosed with multidrug-resistant tuberculosis (MDR-TB) or rifampicin-resistant tuberculosis (RR TB) in 2019. Globally, 206,030 individuals were reported to have MDR-TB/RR TB in 2019, a 10% rise from 186,883 in 2018. Globally, the treatment success rate for MDR-TB/RR TB remains low, at 57%. *(Global Tuberculosis Report 2020).*

Multi-drug-resistant TB (MDR-TB)

MDR tuberculosis is a kind of tuberculosis that is resistant to both isoniazid and rifampicin, the two most effective anti-TB medications. MDR tuberculosis is defined by the World Health Organization (WHO) as resistance to two of the most effective first-line anti-TB medicines (drugs), isoniazid and rifampicin. Drug resistance is one of the most significant difficulties in the treatment of tuberculosis. The primary risk factor for anti-TB medication resistance is prior anti-TB drug therapy, and acquired resistance is a direct and almost immediate consequence of a TB control programme. MDR tuberculosis was also shown to be resistant to a family of medicines known as fluoro quinolones in the majority of patients, both new and previously treated. According to the WHO, around 54% of these patients do not finish therapy and 20% die. Fluoroquinolone resistance is related to a high risk of treatment failure and mortality in an Indian cohort of MDR tuberculosis patients.

TB Care and Prevention

Tuberculosis is curable, even in persons living with HIV. Internationally, DOTS is the preferred approach for tuberculosis control. DOTS therapy employs a range of highly effective antibiotics in a variety of combinations over an extended period to fight germs and assure their eradication. Anti-TB treatment has been found to significantly lengthen the lives of HIV-positive individuals by at least two years. Individuals with the illness must be recognised as soon as feasible so that treatment may begin promptly, contacts can be tracked for tuberculosis examination, and precautions should be taken to limit risk to others. In the majority of instances, tuberculosis is treatable and curable. However, persons with tuberculosis can die if they are not treated properly. DR TB can arise when bacteria develop resistance to the medicines used to treat tuberculosis. *(Global TB Report 2020).*

More than 64 million lives have been saved by the combination of treatment and prevention of TB during the next fifteen years. Globally, there were 7.1 million new TB cases diagnosed and reported in 2019, slightly higher than the 7.0 million diagnosed and reported in 2018 but much higher than the 6.4 million recorded in 2017 and 5.7–5.8 million cases that were observed between 2009 and 2012. For a particular 5-year (2018–2022) goal of reducing the number of TB cases to 40 million, the estimated number of cases this year (2018–2019) has already exceeded 35% of the goal. Almost 14 million. Despite that, there is a notable difference between the number of people who will get diagnosed with TB in 2019 and the number of people who have caught the disease (7.1 million in 2019), with both underreporting and under diagnosis playing a role (either due to lack of access to health care or due to lack of diagnosis. In some cases, even more, severe DR TB may develop. XDR-TB is a form of MDR-TB with additional resistance to more anti-TB drugs. *(India TB Report 2020).*

New WHO Recommendations to Prevent Tuberculosis

World Health Organization (WHO) will assist nations in accelerating efforts to prevent individuals infected with tuberculosis (TB) from becoming unwell by providing preventative treatment. It is believed that one-quarter of the world's population is afflicted with tuberculosis (TB). These individuals are not ill or infectious. They are, nevertheless, more likely to acquire tuberculosis, particularly those with compromised immunity. Giving them TB preventative medication will not only keep them healthy but will also reduce the danger of transmission in the community.

In addition to the commonly used 6 months of daily isoniazid, the WHO proposes novel shorter preventative therapy alternatives. Shorter regimens are currently advised, ranging from a 1-month daily regimen of rifapentine plus isoniazid to 3 months weekly rifapentine plus isoniazid, 3 months daily rifampicin plus isoniazid, or 4 months daily rifampicin alone.

TB prevention is a low-cost strategy that can keep families out of poverty while also protecting the health and economics of entire communities. WHO predicts that when new and safer medications enter the market and prices decline, it will become a very cost-effective approach to save millions of lives.

The Success Rate of MDR-TB Treatment

Globally, 186,772 cases of MDR and RR tuberculosis were identified in 2018, and 156,071patients commenced treatment. MDR-TB has been identified in around 3.4 per cent of new tuberculosis patients and 20% of patients who had previously received tuberculosis therapy globally. In 2019, the WHO updated its MDR tuberculosis treatment recommendations. MDR-TB treatment is lengthy, lasting roughly two years, and involves a combination of numerous second-line medicines that are more costly, less effective, and more hazardous than first-line treatments. As a result, MDR tuberculosis treatment results are dismal, with a success rate of about 54%. MDR/RR tuberculosis treatment success rates remain low globally, at 57 per cent.

Uptake of Diagnostics, New Drugs, and Regimens

Increased access to early and accurate diagnosis through the use of a molecular WHO-recommended fast diagnostic test is one of the primary objectives of the End TB Strategy's laboratory strengthening initiatives. Globally, a WHO-recommended fast diagnostic test detected 2 million patients with tuberculosis (new and relapse) in 2019, accounting for 58 per cent of all bacteriologically proven pulmonary cases. By the end of 2019, 89 countries, primarily in Africa and Asia, had reported using shorter MDR-TB regimens, whereas 86 countries had reported using lengthier all-oral MDR-TB regimens. By the end of 2019, 109 nations have imported or initiated the use of bedaquiline. (Global Tuberculosis Report 2020).

RNTCP in India

The National Tuberculosis Program (NTP) was established by the Government of India in 1962 in the form of a District TB Center model that included BCG vaccination as well as tuberculosis treatment. In the year 1978, The Government of India, the World Health Organization (WHO), and the Swedish International Development Agency (SIDA) conducted a joint review of the National Treatment Programme (NTP) in 1992 and some shortcomings were identified, including managerial weaknesses, inadequate funding, over-reliance on x-ray, non-standard treatment regimens, low rates of treatment completion, and a lack of systematic information on treatment outcomes. At around the same time, in 1993, the World Health Organization (WHO) proclaimed tuberculosis a worldwide emergency, developed the Directly Observed Treatment – Short Course (DOTS) and advised that all nations implement it. DOTS was formally established as part of the RNTCP plan in 1997, and by the end of 2005, the programme had reached every corner of the country.

The Government of India revitalized NTP as the Revised National Tuberculosis Control Programme (RNTCP) was launched by the Indian government in the year 1997. Previously known as the National Tuberculosis Control Programme (NTCP program, DOTS was formally established in 1997 and by the end of 2005, the programme had reached almost all the areas of the country.

India's RNTCP aimed to maintain and enhance a treatment success rate of at least 85% for NSP patients, which included achieving a new case detection rate of at least 85%. It is imperative to have a sensor in place to find 70% of the new sputum-positive individuals who will reside in the neighbourhood. Infected persons who have not previously undergone treatment for TB: Such people are referred to as "new sputum positive" patients. In addition, the TB test has returned a positive result, which classifies the subjects as having the disease.

The RNTCP has been renamed the National Tuberculosis Elimination Program (NTEP) on January 1, 2020. The National Tuberculosis Elimination Program (NTEP) is the Govt. of India's Public Health programme that integrates its anti-tuberculosis activities. It serves as a flagship component of the National Health Mission (NHM) and offers technical and managerial leadership to the country's anti-tuberculosis operations. According to the NSP 2012–17, the initiative seeks to achieve a "TB free India" by Providing Universal Access to TB control services. Through the government health system, the programme delivers a variety of free, high-quality TB diagnostic and treatment services across the country.

Nikshay

NI-KSHAY-(Ni = End, Kshay = TB) is the web-enabled patient management system for TB control under the National Tuberculosis Elimination Programme (NTEP) and allows both public and private sector health care providers to manage their patients. The system that classifies tuberculosis cases in India is called Nikshay. Both public and private healthcare providers use a uniform interface. The accountability of the United DSTB and DRTB relies on the fact that they both proceed through the patient cascade. It eliminates the need for users to enter their user names and passwords each time they desire to access the system. It's simple to use on a mobile device.

NikshayPoshan Yojana (NPY)

The treatment of tuberculosis with nutritional support starting in 2018, the government established the NikshayPoshan Yojana (NPY), a direct benefit transfer initiative to assist those suffering from tuberculosis (TB) with nutritional support. Direct Benefit Transfer programmes were only one of a variety of direct cash transfers benefits transferred to the individual directly (DBT).

Programmatic Management of Drug-Resistant TB (PMDT)

The phrase "Programmatic Management of Drug-Resistant Tuberculosis" (PMDT), formerly known as Directly Observed Treatment, Short-Course (DOTS) Plus, refers to MDR-TB diagnosis, management, and treatment that takes place inside a programme. India began delivering multi-drug-resistant tuberculosis (MDR-TB) diagnostic and treatment services in 2007, and in 2013 it achieved complete coverage. 1.39.369 people were diagnosed with MDR-TB/RR TB in 2016 and 1.26.136 (91%) with RNTCP treatment. The WHO suggested in May 2016 that drug-resistant TB will be much improved, including the provision of shorter schemes to a large number of patients. In the past, the treatment of drug-resistant TB sometimes required the administration of up to two years of a huge number of medications. Furthermore, medications often have significant harmful effects on individuals. As a result, attempts are undertaken to develop shorter, more manageable regimes. It is particularly difficult since it is a two-year treatment scheme with eight months of daily injections and a total of over 14,600 swallowable pills, as well as the fact that a lot of the medicine utilised has risky side effects including sadism, insanity and acute nausea. This has a harmful influence on the psychological & social well-being of individuals with MDR-TB.

Elimination of Tuberculosis in India

Multidrug-resistant tuberculosis (MDR-TB) is another emerging threat to tuberculosis eradication, resulting from an inadequate or deteriorating tuberculosis control programme. The globe has just two cases of tuberculosis per million people when the term "eradication" is used to describe a situation, according to certain estimates. Because of the massive amount of work previously completed, TB elimination in India will not be completed until 2025. The Government of India stated in March 2017 that the country's new tuberculosis goal was to have the disease eradicated by 2025. To achieve our objective of eliminating tuberculosis by 2025, the government will need to adopt a new strategy, approach the problem from a new perspective, and be more aggressive in our efforts. TB is the leading cause of death in the world.

Is MDR-TB is Problem to the Community

MDR-TB, commonly known as drug-resistant tuberculosis, is a major threat to global public health, particularly in low and middle-income countries. Most of the development of MDR-TB is attributable to ineffective clinical outcomes and suboptimal regimen adherence. Approximately 50% of MDR-TB patients fail to complete treatment (WHO). Prolonged treatment length (usually 24 months or longer) and drug toxicity contribute to treatment adherence problems and result in such poor outcomes. A prolonged and thorough treatment plan includes powerful medications that can result in a variety of mental health issues, including psychosis. It has a higher rate of follow-up loss and worse cure outcomes than drug-sensitive tuberculosis, as well as a higher case fatality rate (TB). Other components of psychological ill-health, which are not often addressed, are left to fester and grow. Globally, fewer than half of MDR-TB patients complete their treatment. A significant major reason for these poor outcomes is the lengthy treatment period (which is generally 24 months or longer) and drug toxicity, which results in poor adherence to treatment. Psychological issues are also known to aggravate MDR-TB in some cases. People with multidrug-resistant tuberculosis (MDR-TB) have difficulty finding effective treatment alternatives, as there are just a few treatments, they have to continue treatment for a long time, and the treatments themselves are toxic. Despite advancements in microbiological and clinical research into MDR-TB, psychosocial aspects of the illness are limited and poorly understood.

Scope and Importance of Treating MDR-TB

Numerous studies in India and across the world have shown that MDR-TB patients experience considerable psychological issues with the disease and its treatment effects. There is a very little book investigating the psychological well-being of MDR-TB patients. However, these findings need to be expanded urgently to develop more data that can be utilised to investigate and understand the psychological well-being of MDR-TB patients. A psychosocial intervention model must be set up for MDR-TB patients and their caregivers based on the theory of social work, methodologies and models (strategies). In this academic research, the investigators seek to examine the psychological well-being of MDR-TB patients.

The academic research was conceived because MDR tuberculosis is a significant impediment to attaining the RNTCP's END TB 2025 goal. Tuberculosis medication resistance has the potential to become a significant public health concern in India. As a result, it is critical to monitor treatment adherence, patient well-being, and Loss to Follow-Up (LFU) to assist the patient and the programme. Resistance to medicines used to treat tuberculosis (TB), particularly multidrug-resistant tuberculosis (MDR-TB), has become a serious public health concern in several countries, including India, and is also a barrier to successful tuberculosis control. MDR tuberculosis (MDR-TB) is a major obstacle to worldwide tuberculosis control.

Even though tuberculosis is preventable and treatable, it has surpassed HIV as the most infectious disease killer on the planet. MDR-TB has been designated a "global public health problem" by the WHO and eradicating it will need increased efforts in prevention, diagnosis, and treatment. MDR-TB eradication is a focal point of discussion in the United Nations General Assembly's September high-level conference dedicated to ending the worldwide TB pandemic. There is a dearth of information on the psychological well-being of MDR-TB patients even though only a few studies have examined these emotional and behavioural problems in TB and MDR-TB patients from a clinical and social viewpoint.

This book aims to study MDR-TB patients' treatment experiences, family support, institutional support, physiological distress, stigma and discrimination, and overall health to understand their perspective.

The goal of this study was to assess the Psycho-Social Well-being of MDR-TB patients who live in and was undergoing MDR-TB treatment in Greater Chennai Corporation (GCC) in Tamil Nadu, India. This book seeks to enhance the understanding of the psychological well-being of MDR-TB patients by examining using both quantitative and qualitative data collection methods and using evidence of the patients. The authors emphasizes in his review that TB and multidrug-resistant tuberculosis are linked to psychological distress. Based on this. The authors identified relevant theories, established a theoretical framework, and developed a conceptual framework for the current study. Finally, the findings of this study lean to light on the psychosocial well-being of MDR-TB patients. Furthermore, the study findings also help stakeholders and policy-makers to create and use a sustainable and appropriate social work method for managing MDR-TB.

CHAPTER 2

Psychosocial Well-being of Multi-Drug Resistant Tuberculosis (MDR-TB) Patients

In the previous chapter, the authors presented an overview of the research investigation. In the first chapter, the consequences of tuberculosis and multidrug-resistant Tuberculosis were studied, including the implications and impacts on socioeconomic status, psychological well-being, health, and social stigma. Furthermore, the chapter emphasized the significance of the research topic, the wide-ranging impact of TB and the collateral effects it has on various countries, families, and patients.

This part of the book is an integrated assessment of the available literature on Multidrug-Resistant Tuberculosis (MDR-TB). The book is structured around several perspectives and studies on the topic of MDR-TB and the Psychosocial Well-being of MDR-TB Patients. Through a review of relevant literature, a conceptual framework for psychosocial well-being of MDR-TB patients was developed that is multidimensional and broadly classified into four categories: socioeconomic problems, family and community issues, stigma and discrimination, psychological, medical, and other issues for MDR-TB patients. This framework serves as the foundation for the book's exploration of the Psycho-social Well-being of MDR-TB patients. The chapter begins with a conceptual overview, progresses through key reviews, and concludes with a closing statement. It then moves on to conceptualization and finally to the framework for practice.

This chapter reviews pertinent material and is organised into eight stages. The first stage was a book of pertinent research and literature about the prevalence and extent of tuberculosis. This book begins with an overview of tuberculosis disease, its global effect, regional impact, and impact in India. The second stage is followed by reviews on tuberculosis, which include the history, sources of infection, mode of transmission, tuberculosis and DOTs. The third stage examines the conceptual foundations, prevalence, and magnitude of MDR tuberculosis, followed by a review of MDR tuberculosis treatment and risk factors in the fourth stage. The fifth stage examines the socioeconomic and livelihood consequences of tuberculosis and MDR tuberculosis. The sixth stage involves an evaluation of the stigma associated with tuberculosis and multidrug-resistant tuberculosis by the authors.

Tuberculosis and Multi-Drug Resistant Tuberculosis

The authors conducted a review of related research on tuberculosis, Multi-Drug Resistant Tuberculosis (MDR-TB), Psychological Well-being, General Health, Stigma &Discrimination and MDR-TB management among MDR-TB patients before identifying those related views.

According to a qualitative study conducted in India, MDR-TB has a substantial psychological, social, and economic impact on MDR-TB patients and their families, directly affecting their quality of life. To minimise the harmful consequences of MDR-TB, a psychosocial intervention model (strategies) for MDR-TB patients and their carers are required. (SAARC J TUBER LUNG DIS HIV/AIDS, 2017; XIV, Thiruvalluvan *et al.*).

According to a systematic review conducted in India on Psychological and Economic Issues Facing Multidrug-Resistant Tuberculosis Patients, all studies showed a spectrum of psychosocial and economic difficulties faced by MDR-TB patients. Depression, stigma, discrimination, drug-related side effects causing psychological distress, and financial limitations associated with MDR-TB were also frequently mentioned concerns in the research. There is a paucity of large-scale randomised psychosocial intervention studies that can be scaled up to improve MDR-TB patient treatment, which is critical for the TB control effort. The authors concluded that there is an urgent need to perform research focused on the psychological and socioeconomic components of MDR tuberculosis patients to create evidence. (Isaakidies *et al.*, 2013, India; Morris *et al.*, 2013, Mexico; and Beena Thomas *et al.*, 2016).

Cross-sectional research was conducted on the expenditures spent by MDR-TB patients in the Dominican Republic. The book found that MDR-TB patients had a significant personal financial burden. 2013 Dominican Republic (Mauch *et al.*). Patients experience stigma, prejudice, deliberate separation from their families, loss of self-identity and self-esteem, financial difficulties, and loneliness, according to qualitative research conducted in Mexico. Psychological, social, and economic support treatments should be a routine component of MDR-TB care, according to the authors. Mexico (Morris *et al.*, 2013).

Numerous studies have found that the majority of MDR-TB patients had a perceived loss of self-identity, self-stigma, poor quality of life, low self-esteem, guilt, loneliness, and melancholy (Acha J *et al.*, Peru- 2007, Shin S, Peru-2004; Baral *et al.,* 2014; Lawrence C. Rajkumar and Sathyamurthi K, 2016).

According to research done in Varanasi (India) among Patients with Multidrug-Resistant Tuberculosis, the most prevalent mental diagnosis was depression disorder (28.3 per cent), followed by anxiety disorders (16.7 per cent). This book discovered that MDR-TB patients have considerable psychological distress and mental comorbidity, posing major social and economic problems for their families. The author suggests that MDR-TB patients and their careers require psychosocial support to help minimize the harmful impacts of stigma and manage associated psychological stresses. (2019, Nitesh Kumar *et al.*).

MDR/RR (Rifampicin Resistance) tuberculosis is estimated to account for 3.6 per cent of new cases and 17% of retreatment cases globally. (2018 Report on Global Tuberculosis). On the occasion of World TB Day 2018, India issued its first National Anti-Tuberculosis Drug Resistance Survey (NDRS). The book's major conclusion was that the prevalence of Multi-Drug Resistant Tuberculosis (MDR-TB) was 2.84 per cent and 11.60 per cent, respectively, among new and retreatment TB patients. Additional resistance to fluoroquinolones was seen in 21.82 per cent of patients with MDR-TB (Pre-XDR (Pre-Extensively Drug-Resistant Tuberculosis) with fluoroquinolone resistance). According to state-level statistics, Maharashtra has the highest rate of MDR-TB among new tuberculosis patients (7.72 per cent), significantly higher than the national rate of 2.8 per cent.

Similarly, Uttarakhand had the highest rate of multidrug-resistant tuberculosis among previously treated tuberculosis patients (20%), above the national rate of 15%. (11.62 per cent.) (G.P. Mishra, J.D. Mulani, *et al.*, 2018).

Tuberculosis (TB) is a disease caused by germs that are spread from person to person through the air. It usually affects the lungs, but it can also affect other parts of the body, such as the brain, the kidneys, or the spine. A person with TB can die if he does not get treatment (Centers for Disease Control and Prevention, U.S, 2012). Tuberculosis is a chronic infectious and communicable granulomatous disease caused by mycobacterium tuberculosis (Reza, 2010).

The tubercle bacilli establish infection in the lungs after they are carried in droplets small enough (5 to 10 microns) to reach the alveolar spaces. If the defence system of the host fails to eliminate the infection, the bacilli proliferate inside alveolar macrophages and eventually kill the cells. The infected macrophages produce cytokines and chemokines that attract other phagocytic cells, including monocytes, other alveolar macrophages, and neutrophils, which eventually form a nodular granulomatous structure called the tubercle. If the bacterial replication is not controlled, the tubercle enlarges and the bacilli enter local draining lymph nodes. This leads to lymphadenopathy, a characteristic clinical manifestation of primary tuberculosis (Wani, 2013).

Source of TB Infection

There are two sources of TB infection: human and bovine (connected with domestic and wild mammals). The most common source of infection is human cases whose sputum is positive for tubercle bacilli and who have either received no treatment or have not been treated fully (Park, 2003). Amongst the members of the mycobacterium tuberculosis complex (MTBC), mycobacterium tuberculosis is mainly a human pathogen, whereas Mycobacterium bovis has a broad host range and is the principal agent responsible for tuberculosis (TB) in domestic and wild mammals. Mycobacterium bovis also infects humans, causing zoonotic TB through ingestion, inhalation and, less frequently, by contact with mucous membranes and broken skin.

Zoonotic TB is indistinguishable clinically or pathologically from TB caused by M. tuberculosis (Rua-Domenech, 2006).

In addition, the causative agent of bovine tuberculosis, Mycobacterium Bovis is also responsible for some cases of tuberculosis in human beings. Infection of human beings with Mycobacterium Bovis almost always occurs by inhalation of aerosols or consumption of milk containing the bacillus. Although milk was the usual source of infection for town dwellers, it was considered likely that farm workers were often infected by Mycobacterium Bovis by inhalation and acid-fast bacilli were seen in dried bovine sputum on the walls and windows of cowsheds (Grange, 2001).

Multi-Drug Resistance TB

MDR tuberculosis is caused by Mycobacterium tuberculosis strains that are resistant to at least ionised and rifampicin, two of the most effective first-line anti tuberculosis medicines (Migliori, D'Arcy Richardson, *et al.,* 2009). Molecular epidemiological methods have established that the M. tuberculosis strain dubbed "Beijing" is responsible for MDR-TB epidemics in areas with low tuberculosis prevalence, such as the United States (Drobniewski, Balabanova, *et al.* (2005). Apart from the disease's worldwide danger, it can also result in the more lethal widely drug-resistant tuberculosis (XDR-TB). XDR-TB is caused by Mycobacteria that satisfy all of the criteria for MDR-TB but are also resistant to any fluoroquinolone and at least one of three anti-TB injectable drugs: capreomycin, amikacin, or kanamycin (Migliori, D'Arcy Richardson *et al.* (2009). As might be predicted, both of these types of tuberculosis have a significant death rate. Mortality rates among XDR-TB patients are comparable to those observed in the pre-antibiotic period (Ershova, Kurbatova *et al.* (2012).

MDR-TB and XDR-TB can develop for a variety of causes. To begin, it might be a result of the suppliers. They may recommend insufficient medication regimens for patients, whether it be insufficient dosages, insufficient medicines, incorrect drugs, or insufficient duration of treatment.

The second explanation might be that individuals are not adhering to their recommended medication regimens. Thirdly, the medicines used to treat tuberculosis may be substandard (Migliori, D'Arcy

Richardson, *et al.* (2009). MDR-TB and XDR-TB can be acquired or acquired. Primary drug resistance occurs when MDR-TB or XDR-TB is transferred directly from one person to another. Acquired drug resistance can occur as a result of improper usage of tuberculosis medications. (D'Arcy Richardson, Migliori, *et al.* (2009).

The problem of tuberculosis medication resistance became apparent immediately after streptomycin was introduced in 1944. The British Medical Research Council reported the first fatality from a drug-resistant strain of tuberculosis in 1948. This resulted in the late 1940s discovery of the efficacy of combination therapy with streptomycin and para-aminosalicylic acid against developing drug-resistant bacteria. The length of this therapy regimen, on the other hand, was significantly prolonged. From 1952 through the 1980s, the introduction of INH, RIF, EMB, and PZA kept the situation under control. However, in the early 1990s, multiple outbreaks of MDR-TB, notably among HIV-infected individuals, pushed this disease to the forefront as a serious worldwide public health issue.

Treatment of DR TB and MDR-TB

There is a long and expensive procedure involved in treating DR-TB, and it can take two years to treat using medicines that are less powerful and more toxic than the ones used to treat TB, according to Jenkins, Zignol, and colleagues (2011). The TB treatment plan is based on the patient's precise medications of resistance. Second-line drugs such as rifabutin, ethionamide, prothionamide, Para-amino salicylic acid, D-cycloserine, and thiacetazone are also used. Many different treatments ranging from three to many different medicines may be given at the same time, and treatment may continue from six months to over two years. These three individuals—Ahmad, Suhail, and the others (2010). Care must be taken to monitor patients for compliance with the treatment plan. In the therapy's case, the results will rely on whether the patient has medication resistance if available treatments are listed, and on the patient's participation in the treatment. Simply the best, D'Arcy Richardson, and his collaborators (2009).

Sometimes, in severe situations, the diseased lung tissue has been surgically removed to treat the infection. In patients with significant drug resistance and poor postoperative expectations for lung function, and in the event of a TB drug level that ensures normal healing of the surgical stump, this treatment approach is utilised. Once pharmaceutical treatment has been attempted for at least three months, surgical interventions can be considered, Migliori, D'Arcy Richardson *et al.* (2009). Under DOTS, low-cost diagnosis and treatment of diseases are offered to the public in India.

Risk Factors for MDR-TB

Tuberculosis (TB) medications were accessible in the 1950s, and this coincided with a drop in TB incidence in the West. However, the rise of the human immunodeficiency virus (HIV) allowed the emergence of tuberculosis, and acquired immunodeficiency syndrome (AIDS) ensued (AIDS). 12-14 million individuals are coinfected with HIV and TB as of 2009, as estimated by Shenoi *et al.* HIV individuals are more likely to be infected with tuberculosis (Shenoi, Heysell, *et al.* (2009).

TB patients' peak earning years seem to coincide with the years in which they suffer from the disease, according to research conducted by Nhlema *et al.*, Kamolratanakul, and Rajeswari *et al.* The time it takes a person to obtain necessary treatment, as well as the cost of getting it, are typically higher for the poor. Authorss Nehlma, *et al.* (2003) and Kemp, *et al.* (2007) discovered that impoverished individuals have considerably larger proportions of their income go to paying for medical expenses. Although their total financial outlay is probably less, their relative costs for medical services are much higher.

A survey was conducted by Casal (2005) across Western Europe and found that several risk variables, including immigration, ageing, HIV infection, population movement, living in communities, and drug misuse, were present in nations throughout Europe.

In the book, Dahlgren and Whithead (2006) found that out-of-pocket healthcare expenses can lead to spiralling poverty for many families, and this may put a particularly large burden on the already-impoverished person. In this instance, the phrase "medical poverty trap" has been applied.

Individuals infected with HIV are more prone to other types of tuberculosis (otherwise known as "regular" and "multi-drug resistant") as well as "emerging" and "extensively drug-resistant" tuberculosis. Resistance to tuberculosis medication is commonly linked to the absorption problems associated with HIV/AIDS, which may contribute to greater levels of resistance. They have demonstrated that drinking coffee may help you concentrate more (2010). The results of a cross-country, country-wide book in Estonia show that people with HIV are three times more likely to get the disease.

Socio-Economic Impact

In general, the lower socioeconomic position is associated with poorer health. Tuberculosis is often thought to be a disease of the impoverished and socially marginalised. M.H. Rahman and A. Singh (2011). Because those with lower means typically live in smaller places with more people dwelling in the restricted area, a recognised risk for transmission of highly infectious disease, socioeconomic status is partially connected to the environment. Poorer levels of education are linked to lower incomes and poverty. Z. Oxaal, Z. Oxaal, Z. Oxaal, Z (1997). Poverty and inequality are connected to the incidence of tuberculosis, according to Muniyandi M, *et al.* (2008).

Tuberculosis mostly affects economically active populations in impoverished nations such as India, and as a result, it can have far-reaching economic and social implications for those who are affected, as well as their families and communities (WHO, Stop TB Initiative 2000 series). TB affects the most productive age group, resulting in a high economic burden for society, with patients incurring other direct and indirect costs such as transportation, hospitalisation, and reduced working hours, even though the national tuberculosis programme provides free diagnostic and treatment services to all registered patients.

Impact on Livelihood

According to the WHO, the average tuberculosis patient misses three to four months of work and up to 30% of annual household wages. Income loss due to tuberculosis is estimated to be over $12 billion in the world's poorest areas. According to the World Bank, the loss of productivity due to tuberculosis amounts to 4–7 per cent of certain nations' GDP. T.P. Soubbotina (2004) and M. Muniyandi *et al.*

(2008). McIntyre D., *et al.* (2006) found in their book that there is rising evidence of households being driven into poverty or coerced into deeper poverty when faced with significant medical costs, particularly when paired with a loss of household income due to bad health. Russell S. (2004) discovered in his book that the expense burden of tuberculosis is more than 10% of annual household income; it will be disastrous for the household.

The financial toll on families is, also considerable. TB treatment is frequently free, at least for drug-sensitive tuberculosis, but patients pay extra expenditures, such as transportation and hospital fees, at the same time they have likely curtailed or ceased working entirely. According to the WHO, the average tuberculosis patient misses three to four months of work and up to 30% of yearly household wages.

CHAPTER 3

General Health and the Quality of Life of TB Patients

Generally, medicine is applied more technically and mechanically nowadays, and on the other hand, an effort is required not only for illness control but also for improving patients' quality of life. Quality of life (QOL), defined as an individual's impression of his or her physical and mental health, encompasses a wide range of dimensions, including physical, psychological, social, and environmental well-being. The World Health Organization defines health as a full condition of physical, mental, and social well-being, not only the absence of sickness or disability.

Chow SP, Yau A. (1980) found that physical functioning represents the patient's ability to carry out fundamental day-to-day activities in research on Tuberculosis of the Knee with a long-term follow-up.

In their book, Liefooghe R., Michiels N., Habib S., *et al.* (1995) claimed that psychological health considers various characteristics of an individual's mood and emotional well-being. The WHO guideline Addressing Poverty in TB Control (2005) identifies four types of obstacles to care: geographical, social/cultural, health system, and economic barriers. The three major categories of expenses are 1) health-care charges, 2) transportation, lodging, and sustenance, and 3) missed income, productivity, and time. All of the expected domains of TB, such as general health perception, corporal sense, psychological health, mental peace, and functioning of physical and social duties, have an impact on quality of life.

In research done in Pakistan on socio-cultural limitations in treatment, Khan *et al.* (2008) discovered that while both male and female TB patients experience social and economic issues, female patients are more affected.

Meera Dhuria *et al.* (2008), in their book Impact of Tuberculosis on the Quality of Life, compared the QOL scores in TB patients with those in the general population, finding that TB patients had lower mean scores than controls, with the physical domain being the worst affected, followed by the psychological domain.

In their book, Unalan *et al.* (2008) claimed that QOL is distorted in both active and inactive TB cases and that demographic-sociocultural variables, depression, daily sleep time, treatment period, and concomitant illnesses are factors that impact QOL. When it comes to accepting the TB/MDR-TB diagnosis, patients are frightened, irritated, or disappointed; the economic weight of the disease, as well as the misery of transmitting the disease to others, is also a reason leading to psychological issues. Social functioning refers to a patient's interactions with others at home, work, and in society. Patients are frequently isolated, which causes them to feel lonely, bored, restricted, or abandoned. The environmental element includes MDR-TB patients' living conditions and well-being.

Stigma and Tuberculosis

Stigma, it is frequently stated, is a mark of shame that distinguishes an individual. According to the Mental Health Commission of Australia, when a person is classified according to their condition, they are categorised into a stereotyped group. Negative attitudes breed prejudice, which in turn results in negative behaviour and discrimination. Stigma, in general, results in experiences and sentiments of guilt, blame, misery, hopelessness, and distortion in the media, as well as a reluctance to seek and/or accept required assistance from others. Stigma also affects the patient's family, resulting in a lack of support. To mental health practitioners, stigma implies that patients are seen as aberrant, corrupt, or wicked and that psychotherapeutic therapies are frequently viewed with mistrust and dread.

Irving Goffman classified stigma into three categories: character, physical, and group connection. Character stigmas are labels applied to individuals based on certain aspects of their personalities. Typically, these forms of stigma are determined by a shared set of moral standards that serves as a yardstick for the character in society. Physical stigma is a label applied to individuals based on their appearance. It is considered that physical deformity and odd looks are instances of physical stigma. A group affiliation stigma is a form of discrimination against individuals based on their membership in an existing group. This may be a religion, an ethnic group, or even a political party. Goffman asserts that group affiliation is typically associated with entire families and is carried down generationally.

Baral *et al.* (2007) examine the stigma and prejudice related to tuberculosis in their book. In poor nations, the primary impact is the social isolation of patients, both outside the family, where former friends and acquaintances may shun the individual, and inside the family, where the patient may be compelled to eat and sleep apart. Patients frequently isolate themselves to avoid spreading infection and to avoid unpleasant situations such as being ostracised or being the topic of rumour. Being a patient or an ex-patient will almost certainly have an impact on work and job prospects. Unmarried women may face discrimination from prospective spouses and in-laws, while married women may find themselves divorced owing to tuberculosis or if a family history of tuberculosis is later disclosed.

According to Baral *et al.* (2007), stigma and subsequent discrimination have a dual effect on tuberculosis control. To begin, fear of being recognised as a person with tuberculosis makes it more difficult for people who have a persistent cough and believe they may have tuberculosis to seek care, due to the public nature of the tuberculosis testing procedure. By delaying treatment, these individuals may acquire more significant symptoms, making them more difficult to treat; moreover, since they stay infectious for a longer period, they increase their chances of transmitting the disease to others. Second, worries about stigma and prejudice associated with tuberculosis make it more difficult for patients to maintain care since their fear of being identified as having or having been infected with tuberculosis restricts their daily access to services. This, once again, can result in severe symptoms and increased transmission.

D. Somma *et al.* (2008) examined the indicators of tuberculosis-related stigma as well as sociocultural and gender-related characteristics of disease linked with stigma in Bangladesh, India, Malawi, and Colombia. The authorss discovered that India had the highest overall stigma score, Malawi had the lowest, and Bangladesh had the highest for women. Women were more concerned about the influence on their marriage chances in India and Malawi. Associations with HIV/AIDS were found to be associated with TB stigma in Malawi, where sexual contact as a perceived cause was more associated with stigma for men and less associated with stigma for women, concluding that stigma both influences and indicates the effectiveness of tuberculosis control. Cultural epidemiological approaches shed light on the universal and local characteristics of stigma and gender in the context of tuberculosis control.

Psychosocial Well-being and Psychological Distress

Coping with and overcoming life's difficulties are more of a norm than an exception. According to Iseman (1993), treating MDR-TB is more challenging than treating drug-sensitive TB, because second-line TB medicines are more difficult to get, frequently need intravenous administration, and are more toxic and ineffective than first-line TB treatments. Additionally, Booker (1996) noted that MDR-TB treatment might take up to two years or longer, resulting in social isolation, job loss, and long-term socioeconomic and psychological consequences. Numerous individuals are impacted at any one moment by acute and chronic diseases, accidents, and disasters of various types, as well as issues linked to crime, delinquency, the HIV/AIDS pandemic, drug addiction, and alcoholism (Levine & Perkins, 1997). Ormerod (2007) discovered that individuals with multidrug-resistant tuberculosis (MDR-TB) are resistant to either ionised (INH) or rifampin, or both medications. Additionally, patients with MDR-TB require longer, more expensive treatment regimens and have a greater death rate than those with drug-sensitive tuberculosis.

Psychological Distress and Tuberculosis

Psychological distress is a broad word that describes sensations or emotions that impair one's ability to operate normally. To say that it is the psychological discomfort that interferes with your daily activities is to state that this discomfort gets in the way of your regular activities. Depression and negativity about the environment, others, and the self are common results of psychological suffering. Though emotions such as sorrow, worry, and distraction are commonly associated with mental illness, they are only symptoms. Thus, no two people have the same perspective when viewing an event. Psychological anguish is an individual experience, regardless of what others say. Psychological discomfort is impacted by the circumstances and our perception of it. "Mental health" and "mental disease" are opposite ends of a spectrum that describes the level of psychological suffering someone experiences.

Feeling about Infectious Diseases Like TB

Many studies have revealed that patients with mycobacterial illnesses might have a wide range of symptoms including reduced appetite, fever, cough. In other situations, no symptoms are present, the disease is identified. Each of these circumstances has various problems. There is typically worry and misunderstanding surrounding new symptoms in patients with numerous symptoms. What's wrong with me? What's wrong? Why don't I normally do the things I do? Am I going to be all right? It might be a shock to be notified of a severe condition that requires long-term care in individuals with no symptoms if they feel well. The patient can hardly think that the tests/diagnosis for them are correct.

When a diagnosis is made, it is common to have feelings of fear, shock, denial, anger, shame, and guilt, among other things. These feelings may come in waves, and they will progressively fade over time as the patient receives a therapeutic reduction of symptoms. When it comes to infectious diseases, shame is likely to be experienced more often than in other chronic diseases, as is the requirement of wearing a mask and being temporarily protected from contagious disorders such as infectious diseases. Furthermore, precautions are made to prevent the spread of the infection. Solitude may be one of the most difficult aspects of the illness. Patients have a tough time dealing with the feelings of being dirty or ostracized. In general, the more someone feels, the better they can cope with the situation. Even with support, though, it may be extremely difficult and uncomfortable to wear a mask and be isolated from other people for long periods.

Effects on Relationships and Self Esteem

Additionally, worries of death or permanent incapacity may arise, as well as concerns about the drugs and their probable adverse effects, as well as concerns about lifestyle changes. As noted in socio-economic research on tuberculosis, individuals may be unable to work, resulting in financial hardship for themselves and their families. Relatives and friends may be fearful of the diagnosis and may struggle for a while to be supportive. Additionally, illness frequently necessitates a shift in one's interpersonal ties. The patient may become significantly more reliant on others. Being even a little dependant on a patient who is extremely self-sufficient can be quite unpleasant.

Patients may feel guilty, angry, or depressed; family members and friends may also feel these emotions. To adapt to the illness's demands, an extraordinary level of flexibility is required. It is critical to find strategies to preserve a healthy level of independence. What becomes critical is preserving one's self-esteem while coping with a chronic disease that presents obstacles and problems.

Depression and Anxiety

Clinical investigations on tuberculosis have shown that the stress of having a chronic illness can be significant, resulting in mental anguish. You may feel melancholy or worried at times. When our lives are severely disturbed, we frequently feel emotional distress. Mycobacterial illness symptoms might include weakness, exhaustion, lack of appetite and energy, and shortness of breath, all of which are signs of depression or anxiety.

Clinical trials and research have shown that several medicines used to treat mycobacterial infections can affect emotional functioning, causing agitation or disorientation. It might be difficult to distinguish between the many causes of sadness and anxiety. It may necessitate the collaboration of family members, physicians and nurses, and, in certain cases, a psychosocial clinician. Emotional discomfort is quite prevalent in the short term. When depression or anxiety is severe or protracted, it can lead to additional impairment and interfere with therapeutic progress.

Several writers discovered frequent comorbidity of tuberculosis with common mental illnesses, including Trenton AJ (2001) and Yang L, *et al.* (2003). Few studies have looked at prevalent mental illnesses in TB patients in low and middle-income countries (LMICs), and they have discovered a significant prevalence of CMDs in Pakistan, ranging from 46.3 to 80%. Hussain MO, *et al.* (2008) and Aamir SA, (2010), Nigeria 27.7 to –30%, Issa BA, *et al.* (2009), and Aghanwa HS *et al.* (1998), Ethiopia 64% Deribew A, *et al.* (2010), India 76% Prakash C, *et al.* (2011), South Africa 46%, Westaway MS *et al.* (1992), Naidoo P, *et al.* (2010), and Turkey 19–26% IO Aydin *et al.* (2001).

Male gender Sulehri MA, *et al.* (2010), adverse effect on drug compliance and TB treatment gender Sulehri MA, *et al.* (2010), low educational attainment, financial status, no source of income in day labourers, an increase in the number of symptoms reported, more serious perceived consequences, and less control over their illness, in TB/HIV co-iDeribew A, *et al.* (2010), and Duarte EC, *et al.* (2009), older age groups, the young and the elderly, Issa BA, *et al.*, (2009), and Aghanwa HS *et al.*, (1998), and poor TB treatment result (death) Kessler R, *et al.* (2002).

In his study on Common mental disorders (CMDs), which include depression, anxiety, and somatoform disorders, Siddiqi K *et al.*, (2007) found that they contribute significantly to the burden of disease and disability in low- and middle-income countries (LMICs) (WHO, Mental Health new understanding new hope, 2001). These diseases are responsible for up to 10% of all illnesses worldwide. CMDs affect at least one-third of all patients seen in LMIC primary care settings. The bulk of these patients' burdens have CMDs that are not recognised nor adequately addressed. Even though depression and anxiety disorders are listed as independent diagnostic categories in the WHO's ICD-10 Geneva Report 2007, they are not. Because of the significant degree of co-morbidity between these diseases in primary care, as well as the similarities in epidemiological profiles and treatment responsiveness, the notion of CMDs is relevant for public health initiatives, according to Patel V *et al.* (2009).

CHAPTER 4

Theoretical Perspective and Models of Tuberculosis

In this chapter of the book, it deals about the various perspectives of tuberculosis and multi drug resistant tuberculosis.

Biomedical Perspective

The biomedical perspective integrates biomedical theory, which assumes that patients are passive receivers of physicians' instructions. Because health and sickness are linked back to biological factors such as germs or viruses, therapy is directed towards the patient's body (Ross F., Deverell A: Psychosocial approaches to health, illness and disability: A reader for health care professionals. 2004). Mechanical remedies, such as prescription medications, are favoured under this mechanistic perspective of sickness; non-adherence is thought to be caused by patient attributes such as age and gender (Blackwell B, Compliance, Psychotherapy and psychosomatics, 1992). Technological advancements aimed at improving adherence, such as Medication Event Monitoring Systems, are frequently based on this approach (WHO, Adherence to long-term therapies, Evidence for action. Geneva, 2003) However, despite the implicit use of this perspective by a substantial number of health care professionals, it is rarely used explicitly in clinical practice.

Behavioural (learning) Perspective

This perspective combines behavioural learning theory (BLT), which places a premium on the environment and the training of adherence-management skills. It is defined by the application of the antecedents and consequences concepts, as well as their effect on behaviour. The antecedents might be internal (thoughts) or external (environmental signals), and the consequences can be either penalties or incentives for the behaviour. The likelihood that a patient will engage in a certain behaviour will be influenced by these variables (WHO, Adherence to long-term therapies, Evidence for action. Geneva, 2003).

Communication Perspective

According to the Institute of Medicine, communication is the "cornerstone of every patient-practitioner interaction." This viewpoint implies that enhanced provider-client communication will result in increased adherence. (World Health Organization, Adherence to long-term therapies: Evidence of effectiveness. Geneva, 2003, and (Ross E, Deverell A: Psychosocial approaches to health, illness, and disability: A reader for health care professionals. 2004) imply that this can be accomplished through patient education and effective health care worker communication skills – an approach predicated on the premise that communication must be clear and understandable in order to be effective., also emphasises the importance of treatment timing. An intervention utilising this approach, for instance, attempts to enhance client-provider contact. According to critics of this approach, it overlooks attitudinal, motivational, and interpersonal elements that may obstruct the message's receipt and translation into behaviour change. B. Blackwell (1992).

Cognitive Perspective

Theories in the cognitive viewpoint include the health belief model (HBM), social-cognitive theory (SCT), theories of reasoned action (TRA) and planned behaviour (TPB), and the protective motive theory (PMT). These theories emphasise cognitive factors as part of behaviour change and share the idea that attitudes and beliefs, Stroebe W (2000), as well as expectations of future events and results, Gebhardt WA and Maes S (2001), are important predictors of health-related behaviour. These theories argue that in the face of several options, people will select the action that is most likely to result in favourable consequences.

Health Belief Model

The Health Belief Model (HBM) is a psychological model which seeks to explain and predict health behaviour. This is done through identifying and addressing the personal attitudes and beliefs of participants. In the 1950s, public health psychologists Hochbaum, Rosenstock, and Kegels of the U.S. Public Health Service created the HBM to help psychoanalysts assess patients with mental illnesses. it perceives behaviour modification as being based on a sober assessment of the disparity between the blocks to and rewards of action (Blackwell B, Compliance, Psychotherapy and psychosomatics, 1992).

This model proposes that individuals' perception of their own and their families' threat of sickness is determined by their perceptions of the seriousness of and vulnerability to disease. In essence, perceptions of the positive and negative effects of certain health behaviours have the same impact on perceived efficacy. People's subjective view of the chances of success as well as the perceived urgency of the problem has a direct impact on how seriously people see the situation. The perceived danger is affected by a stimulus that encourages an action, whether it's internal (e.g., symptom perception) or external (e.g., triggers) (e.g., health communication). Authorss in Redding, California, and elsewhere, (2000) and WHO, found that adherence to long-term treatments helps people get well.

The Protection-Motivation Theory

According to this theory, changing an individual's behaviour may be accomplished by appealing to their anxieties. Three components of fear arousal are postulated: the amount of damage associated with a portrayed event; the likelihood of that event occurring; and the efficacy of the protective reaction, Rogers RW (1975). These, it is said, interact multiplicatively to determine the degree of protective motivation Stroebe W, (2000), resulting in behaviour motivated by a desire to protect oneself from danger, Rogers RW (1975). This is the only theory within the larger cognitive approach that makes explicit use of the costs and benefits of present and suggested behaviour in predicting the likelihood of change. W.A. Gebhardt & S. Maes (2001).

Social-cognitive Theory

In social-cognitive theory, awareness of health risks and benefits is a requirement for a change; however, there must be additional self-influences to change (Bandura A (2004). Among some of these variables, personal efficacy beliefs play a key part in the transformation. Since the positive and negative effects of the behaviour, financial losses, and benefits on human health will also be included in the predictions, the projected results will alter human health habits. As social results, social acceptance or rejection of a certain activity is another type of social outcome, so too is it the case that social outcomes include these. Results can also be affected by whether or not a person views their health and condition in a favourable or negative light. Additionally, another behaviour factor is facilitators and barriers. Alternatively, this behaviour shift may be caused by the lack of impediments (Bandura A (2004). This idea holds that people act when they feel they have control over the outcome, are prevented from doing anything from the outside, and believe in their ability to carry out the act. These two are made for each other: C.J. and Connor (2000).

This theory emerged from the social theory of learning and might be the most thorough explanation of conduct modification that has been produced up to now (Redding CA *et al.* (2001). In regulating human motivation, action and well-being, it presents a multi-layered causality (and gives both adherence predictors and suggestions for their promotion, Bandura A (2000). The fundamental organisational concept of behavioural change that this theory proposes is mutual determinism in which the connection of the individual, the environment and behaviour continues, and is dynamic (Redding CA *et al.* (2001).

Theory of Planned Behaviour and the Theory of Reasoned Action

The Planed Behaviour's Theory (PLB) was established as the Reasoned Action theory in 1980 to anticipate the purpose of a person to conduct at a certain point in time. The idea was designed to explain all behaviours that people can control themselves. The fundamental element of this paradigm is behavioural intent. The attitude toward the likely result of the behaviour and the subjective appraisal of risks and rewards of it is impacted by the intents of behaviour.

A wide range of health behaviours, including smoking, drinking, use of health services, nursing and drug use, have been effectively predicted and explained via TPB. The TPB asserts that behavioural performance depends on desire and ability (behavioural control). It distinguishes between three kinds of convictions - conduct, norms and control. The TPB consists of six structures that together reflect the real behaviour control of a person.

- **Attitudes:** This term refers to a person's degree of approval or disapproval of certain behaviour. It requires an examination of the behaviour's consequences.
- **Behavioural intention:** This refers to the motivating variables that impact a specific behaviour, with a stronger desire to execute the behaviour increases the likelihood that the behaviour will be completed.
- **Subjective norms:** This relates to an individual's view about whether or not the majority of others approve or disapprove of a particular behaviour. It refers to a person's thoughts regarding whether or not his or her peers and significant others believe the individual should engage in the behaviour.
- **Social norms**: This term refers to the established behavioural rules within a group of individuals or a wider cultural environment. Within a group of individuals, social standards are regarded as normative, or standard.
- **Apparent power:** This relates to the perceived presence of elements that may support or impede the behaviour's performance. Each of those elements contributes to a person's perceived behavioural control.
- **Perceived behavioural control:** This relates to an individual's impression of the ease or difficulty with which they can accomplish the desired behaviour. Perceived behavioural control changes between situations and acts, resulting in a person's impression of behavioural control changing according to the scenario. This construct of the theory was added later and

created the shift from the Theory of Reasoned Action to the Theory of Planned Behavior.

Theoretical Model of Planned Behavior

The TMPB has numerous restrictions, which include the following:

- It presupposes, regardless of intention, that the individual has obtained the opportunity and resources to be effective in doing the desired behaviour.
- It does not take into consideration other factors that influence behavioural intention and motivation, such as fear, anger, mood, or experience.
- While normative variables are included, environmental or economic elements that may impact a person's intention to execute the behaviour are not.
- It believes that behaviour is the product of a linear decision-making process and ignores the possibility of change over time.
- While the addition of the construct of perceived behavioural control was a significant contribution to the theory, it says nothing about real behavioural control.
- The theory does not explain the temporal lag between "intent" and "behavioural action."
- The TPB has shown to be more useful in public health than the Health Belief Model, although it remains constrained by its inability to account for environmental and economic variables. Authorss have used certain TPB elements and added other components from behavioural theory to make it a more integrated model during the last many years. This is a response to some of the TPB's shortcomings in addressing public health issues.
- The theory of reasoned action (TRA) is a paradigm for predicting behavioural intention that includes both attitude and behaviour predictions. Following the separation of behavioural intention from behaviour, it is possible to explain limiting constraints on attitudinal influence (Ajzen, 1980).

Interpersonal Theory

Psychological problems are attributed by interpersonal theories to dysfunctional patterns of interaction (Carson *et al.,* 1996). They stress that we are social creatures and that much of who we are is shaped by our interactions with others. Psychological distress is defined as maladaptive behaviour noticed in relationships that are induced by unsatisfying previous or present relationships. Examining the troubled person's many patterns of interpersonal connections reveals psychological discomfort. According to this viewpoint, pain is eased through interpersonal therapy, which focuses on resolving difficulties within relationships and assisting people in achieving more satisfying relationships through the acquisition of new interpersonal skills.

Erving Goffman Theory of Stigma

These stigmatised people are not fully accepted and continuously strive to change their social identity: physically deformed, mentally deformed, drug-dependent persons, and prostitutes.

Three stigma categories are identified by Goffman: character-related stigma, physical stigma and group identification stigma. The stigma of characteristics is 'singular characteristics which are perceived as weak-will, predatory or unnatural loves, abusive and rigid beliefs and dishonesty, which can be derived from a well-known record such as psychological disorder, imprisonment, dependence, alcoholism, homosexuality, unemployment, suicide and radical political behaviour.' Physical stigma is a reference to bodily physical defects. The stigma of group identification, finally, is a stigma derived from being a certain race, nation, religion, etc.

The social cognitive model is the basis for self-regulatory convictions and behaviours and human ability to be autonomous, Roommaker (2000). Self-efficacy and attributions are two beliefs that govern self-regulatory measures. Self-effectiveness beliefs refer to the confidence of a person in his or her ability to do certain jobs (1997 & 1998). These ideas are essential since there is no desire to act if individuals do not think that they can alter their situation.

This conviction is crucial in health habits so that the client follows the prescription scheme or not. Attributive assumptions are causes for a person's results or accomplishments and as such the assumptions impact behaviour and expectations. Three aspects of assignments are utilised to comprehend the particular reasons one produces for the outcome; locus of causation; stability and controllability. Causality is internal or external (people assign the result to themselves) (attribute outcomes to forces outside themselves). Understanding these convictions can teach caregivers about health sources, including preventative activities, coping behaviours, risk behaviour, compliance and autonomy.

Social Cognitive Perspective

Bandura's (1986, 1997, 1999) social-cognitive paradigm entails the reciprocal links between cognition/personal, behaviour, and environment. These are interdependent causative elements, yet one can have an impact on the others in a reciprocal way. Beliefs about one's competence; reasons for success and failure; and a sense of control, values, and objectives connected to Health and Treatment adherence are examples of cognitive/personal determinants. Environmental variables include a cultural context (society and community), disease exposure (sigma, discrimination,) and social support (Family, Friends, Relatives and Neighbours). Individual behaviour (Psychological Distress, Fear, and Anxiety) encompasses psychosocial well-being and patients' coping strategies. The three components are inextricably linked (i.e., each affects the other).

Because of the prevalence of both physical and social variables among MDR-TB patients, the environment was an essential component. The notion that human thoughts and feelings formed in response to environmental circumstances while also influencing the environment have been the major strength of social cognitive theory (Bandura, 1997). All of these variables were present in the setting of MDR-TB patients' psychological well-being.

Theoretical Framework

The four viewpoints Biomedical, Behavioural, Communication, and Social Cognitive Models were investigated as a method to aid the understanding of the complicated issue of the psychosocial well-being of MDR-TB patients, with diverse cultures from three distinct states of India. Among the cognitive perspectives examined were the health belief model (HBM), social-cognitive theory (SCT), theories of reasoned action (TRA) and planned behaviour (TPB), and protection motivation theory (PMT). Of the aforementioned theories, Social Cognitive Theory (SCT) was most appropriate for the book.

According to Bandura (1998), the social cognitive model describes the methods, resources, and support necessary to modify hazardous behaviour. This section summarises the social cognitive model's fundamental tenets and explains why the authors chose it to guide his understanding of health issues affecting MDR-TB patients, including socioeconomic status, livelihood, stigma and discrimination, quality of life, psychosocial well-being, and psychological distress. Following the examination of these theoretical concerns, a description of the research investigation is provided.

Conceptual Framework

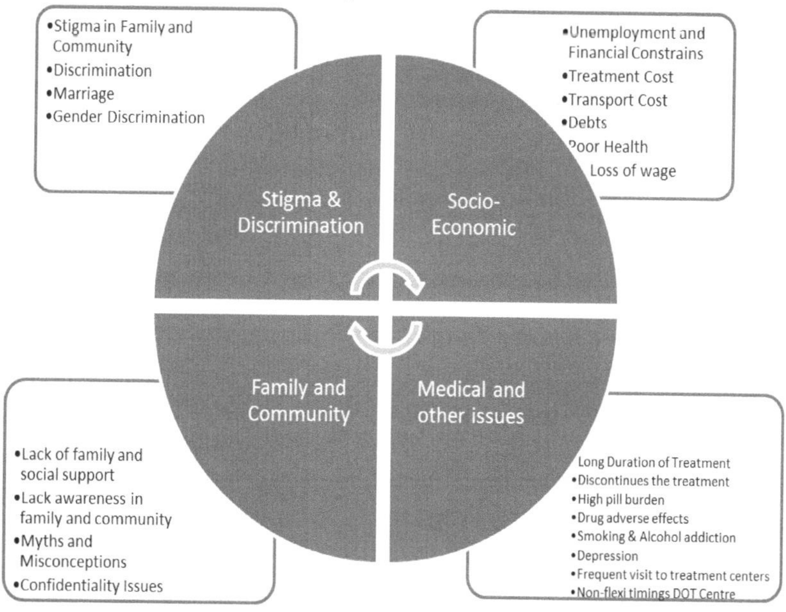

The authors emphasized in his literature review that tuberculosis and multidrug-resistant tuberculosis are associated with psychological distress. Based on the literature survey, field experience, as well as the need and significance of the book, relevant theories were selected, a theoretical framework was constructed, and a conceptual framework was developed for the current research. As per the above conceptual framework and based on the book objectives, the following information was collected from the MDR-TB patients in Chennai corporation.

Personal and Demographic Information

MDR-TB patients' demographic and personal profiles include their age, gender, state, religion, educational status, marital status, family type, and family members. The inclusion of these factors as independent variables is utilised to assess the psychosocial well-being of MDR-TB patients. Each of the demographic profile factors was shown to be favourably associated with this book of MDR-TB patients. As a result, it was chosen to include the aforementioned independent factors in the research.

Socioeconomic Profile

In this book, the socioeconomic profile comprises earning members of the family, Employment Status, Nature of Work, Patient Monthly Income, Total Family Income, Type of House, House Rent Paid, The family has a PDS/Ration Card, as well as a government pension.

Treatment for Tuberculosis and MDR Tuberculosis

The TB treatment history comprises the duration of the TB disease, the patient's past therapy, the location of previous treatment, and the type of previous treatment received. Money spent on private therapy, completion of private treatment MDR-TB treatment length, difficulty with MDR-TB therapy, patient feelings about MDR-TB treatment, money and quantity spent on MDR-TB treatment.

Family Support Profile

The family support of MDR-TB patients contains information about family support during the disease, isolation by family members, sleeping patterns, eating with family members, and use of separate glass and plates.

Institutional Support

The institutional support comprises information on referring a person to the government hospital, the distance to the government hospital, opinions on government hospital treatment, opinions on government hospital staff service, and sources for taking daily DOT.

CHAPTER 5

Materials and Methods of Treating MDR-TB Patients

Introduction

A conceptual framework for the book was developed by the authors after conducting a literature review. Based on this framework, research questions were formulated, and goals were finalized. Aim, objectives, and research design are the subheadings in this Chapter of the book that define the methodology of the book. In addition, the authors have provided information on the subjects of the book, data collection methods and operational definitions, and also book limitations and chapterization.

Area of the Study

The MDR-TB patients in 5 health districts were recruited in Chennai City, South India. The five health districts that were selected for this survey were based on the particular circumstances and treatment facilities available for the patients (Chennai-North, East, West, South, and Central). The capital city of the Indian state of Tamil Nadu is Chennai, also known as Madras. Chennai is one of the biggest cultural, commercial and educational centres in Southern India, located on the Coromandel Coast of the Bay of Bengal. It is India's sixth-most-populated urban centre with the fourth-populated urban agglomeration according to the 2011 census, with a population of 4646732. The Chennai Metropolitan Area is, by population, the 36th biggest metropolitan area in the world. Almost 45 per cent of medical visitors are attracted to Chennai, which is visited by between 30% and 40% of tourists visiting India. It is called the 'Health Capital of India' as such.

The Chennai Corporation is divided into five districts and 15 zones. Chennai has world-class medical facilities, including both public and private institutions. The Chennai Corporation's General Hospital, the TB Sanatorium, the ICMR-National Tuberculosis Research Institute (NIRT), and the Urban Primary Health Centers are all government facilities (UPHC). The RNTCP has been in place in Chennai since 1999. In the RNTCP, there are now 42 TB units and 70 Designated Microscopic Centers (DMC). The number of tuberculosis patients has increased from 7,000 to 8,000 every year. At all Chennai Corporation UPHCs, all TB patients were registered and treated for free for 6 to 8 months. In 2016, 74,782 people were tested for tuberculosis, with 7,990 being diagnosed and receiving treatment. The success rate of anti-tuberculosis therapy is 80%.

The research participants included all MDR-TB patients enrolled in the Chennai corporation TB clinics and DOTS plus centre as part of the updated Revised National Tuberculosis Control Programme (RNTCP). This category was taken into account in the selection of samples in the district. Therefore, all tuberculosis clinics for MDR-TB patients are registered in all five districts of the Chennai Corporation using the census method of sample selection.

Reviews of literature related to psychosocial challenges of MDR-TB patients gave insights regarding the research gaps in the area, helped to identify the research problem and facilitated in developing the conceptual framework on psychosocial challenges of MDR-TB patients. Based on the researchable components of the problem specified in the conceptual framework for psychosocial challenges of MDR-TB patients the research objectives were formulated.

Aim and Objectives of the Research

The General Objective is to understand the Psychosocial Well-being of Multi-Drug Resistance Tuberculosis (MDR-TB) Patients. The Specific Objectives are to study the socio-economic profile, to assess the general health status, to analyse the psychosocial well-being, to understand the stigma & discrimination experienced and to study the support system for MDR-TB patients.

Study Population

Multi-Drug Resistance Tuberculosis (MDR-TB) Patients.

Inclusion Criteria

- Those diagnosed with MDR-TB under the National Tuberculosis Elimination Program (NTEP) within Greater Chennai Corporation (GCC) in five health districts (North Chennai, East Chennai, Central Chennai, West Chennai, and South Chennai) are taking treatment in the Tuberculosis and other urban primary health facilities.
- Those who are aged 18 years and above.
- Those who are willing to take part in the study after the informed consent process have been completed.

Research Design

The research has adopted the descriptive research study design. The research study aimed at describing the background characteristicof persons affected by Multi Drug-Resistant TB and their psycho-social well-being, socio-economic condition, general health status, psychological distress and self-stigma. The authors had adopted thc descriptive research design to explain these background characteristics and explain its relationships with other variables. The study had described the demographic & personal profile of the MDR-TB patients such as Age, Gender, Religion, Educational Status, Marital Status, Children, Family Type, Members in the family, Socio-economic conditions such as earning members in the family, employment status, nature of work, Patient Monthly income, total family income, type of house, the family has PDS/Ration Card.

The TB treatment profiles include the duration of TB illness, patient previous treatment, from where previous treatment was taken, money spent on private treatment etc., and with regard to the MDR-TB treatment that included the details of treatment duration, the problem with the treatment, patient feeling about the treatment, money and amount spent on MDR-TB treatment.

The family support profile includes the details of family support during this illness, isolation by the family members, sleeping pattern, taking food with family members and usage of separate glass and plate. The institutional support profile includes distance to the government hospital, opinion on government hospital treatment, opinion on government hospital staff service and sources of taking daily DOT's. Besides, the research book examines the psychosocial well-being of MDR tuberculosis patients in Chennai Corporation. As a result, the research book focuses on describing the psychosocial characteristics of MDR-TB patients, which serves as a descriptive research design.

Sampling Design

The Universe and Sampling Frame

Study participants are above the age of 18 years undergoing treatment for Multi-Drug Resistant TB forms the universe of book. All MDR-TB patients registered under the Government Revised National Tuberculosis Control Programme (RNTCP) programme and undergoing MDR-TB treatment in 42 Tuberculosis units in Chennai Corporation of their treatment would form the sampling frame of this book.

Map 5.1.1 Greater Chennai Corporation Map showing the 15 Zone

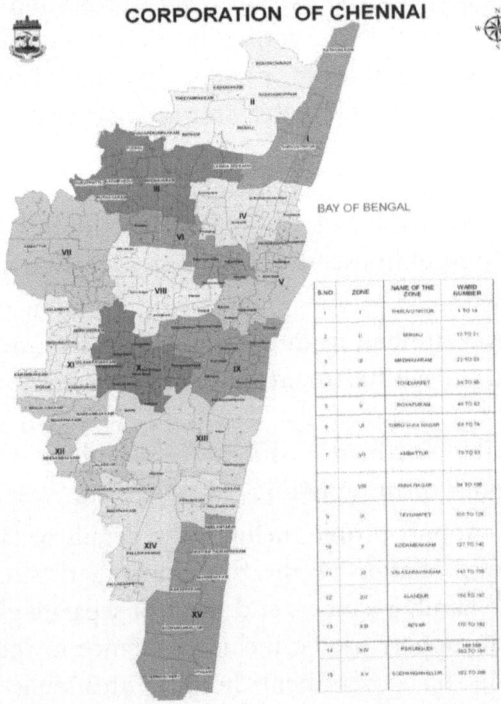

Sample Size

The Census Method was adopted for screening the MDR-TB patients. To fulfil the criteria for the sampling for the census method the following procedure was adopted for sample size selection. A list of patients registered for MDR-TB treatment under the Revised National Tuberculosis Control Programme (RNTCP) in Chennai was received from the District Tuberculosis office. The total number of patients on the list was 323. Out of three hundred and twenty-three MDR-TB patients, the authors removed seven deceased patients, another nineteen who lost to follow up (LFU). Hence the 26 patients were not considered for this study. And finally, two hundred and ninety (297) were eligible for the study. Hence 297 is considered for the sample of the study.

An informed consent form was given to two hundred and ninety-seven (297) MDR-TB patients and requested them to participate in the study. Those who are willing to provide the written informed consent process were completed. Then the interview was conducted in the health facility (TU) itself as per the patient's convenient time. Eight patients were not willing to participate in the study due to their personal and privacy issues. A total of 289 respondents who were willing to participate in the study were enrolled and interviewed.

Table 5.1: Health Districts Wise Sampling Distribution

S. No.	*Name of the Health Districts in Chennai Corporation*	*MDR-TB Patients*	
		Frequency	*Percent*
1.	North Chennai	89	30.8
2.	East Chennai	77	26.6
3.	Central Chennai	59	20.4
4.	West Chennai	36	12.5
5.	South Chennai	28	9.7
Total		**289**	**100**

Table 5.1 shows that the Health Districts wise Sampling Distribution The data has collected from two hundred and eighty-nine (289) MDR-TB patients from 5 Health Districts in Chennai

(North, East, West, South and Central) of Chennai Corporation, those who are diagnosed for MDR-TB and taking treatment under the National Tuberculosis Elimination programme (NTEP) formerly known as the Revised National Tuberculosis Programme. The Sampling Distribution of Multi-Drug Resistant Tuberculosis Patients in Greater Chennai Corporation (GCC). GCC has 15 zones consisting of 200 wards. The expanded Chennai Corporation was divided into three regions—North Chennai, South Chennai and Central Chennai for better administration. Greater Chennai Corporation Health department has decided to divided into 5 health districts (North Chennai, East Chennai, Central Chennai, West Chennai and South Chennai) for the National Tuberculosis Elimination Program (NTEP) in the year 2020 which was formerly known as Revised National TB Control Programme (RNTCP) and strengthen the programme.

Research Method

The authors used a mixed-method design to book the psychological well-being of patients with Multi-Drug Resistant Tuberculosis. The major data collection method used was were interview schedules; tools for psychological well-being, Stigma and Discrimination Scale, and the General Health Questionnaire (GHQ12). Methods of Qualitative Focus Group Discussions were held to have a better understanding of the family and institutional support systems for MDR-TB patients.

Tools for Data Collection

The following are the tools used for primary data collection. The authors used a semi-interview schedule by including the standardized instruments for the specific objectives of the study, and the tools are as follows:

Interview Schedule

This formed the first part of the tool which consists of demographic & personal profiles, such as Age, Gender, Religion, Educational Qualification, Marital Status, Family Type, Number of Family members in the family. The socio-economic profile included the employment status, employment sector, earning members in the family, Monthly income of the MDR-TB patient, Total Family Monthly Income, Earning members in the MDR-TB patients family, Nature of work, patient's monthly income, total family monthly income, Earning members in the MDR-TB patients family, MDR-TB Patients having Public Distribution System (PDS) Ration Card and MDR-TB Patients having Public Distribution System (PDS) Ration Card. Duration of TB illness of MDR-TB Patient, Expenditure made for TB/MDR-TB treatment, from where previous treatment was taken, The problem faced by the MDR-TB patients, MDR-TB patients feeling during treatment.

Family support received by the patients during illness, the feeling of isolation by the MDR-TB patients. sleeping patterns of MDR-TB patients, taking daily food with family members, provided separate glasses and plates to take their food at home by their family members, Distance to Reach Govt. Health Facility from patient's residence, Opinion on Treatment Facility at Government Hospital and Opinion on Government Hospital Staff Service.

Psychological Well-being Scale 42 Item Scale

A 42 item psychological well-being scale was used with Likert scoring to examine the psychological well-being of patients with MDR-TB.

The 12-Item General Health Questionnaire (GHQ-12)

The authorss adopted the General Health Questionnaire (GHQ 12), comprising 12 questions, and adopted the Likert scale, which is a self-administered screening questionnaire designed for use in consulting settings aimed at detecting individuals with a diagnosable psychiatric disorder. This tool was used by the authorss to collect data on general health to assess the evidence of psychological distress among MDR-TB patients.

Internalized Stigma of Mental Illness (ISMI) Scale

The authorss adopted the Internalised Sigma of Mental Illness (ISMI) scale, which consists of 28 questions. The first part of the 6 questions focused on alienation (patient separation), the next part from questions

7 to 12 includes stereotype (labelling) endorsements, the questions from 13 to 23 included discrimination experiences of the patients, and lastly, questions 24 to 28 include stigma resistance.

Focus Group Discussion

The authors conducted 5 focus group discussions (FGD) by using the interview guide with MDR-TB patients, to study the support systems of patients to understand and triangulate with Quantitative Research Method.

Pilot Study

The authors conducted a pilot study in which they were visited TB units and interacted with the RNTCP Health Visitor, MDR-TB Co-Ordinator's, STS and STLS, and other officials from each of the TB units in the 5 Health Districts in Chennai, as well as the DOTS plus site where MDR-TB patients are admitted for observation during the treatment initiation. The authors talked with the patients about their health problems and the impact they were having on their lives. This helped the authorss gain a better understanding of the patients' health problems and related issues, which helped the authors become more familiar with the health-related issues of MDR-TB patients.

Sources of Data

The Primary Data

The sources of data collection for the book on the Psychosocial Well-being of Multi-Drug Resistant Tuberculosis (MDR-TB) Patients are classified as primary and secondary. The primary data were collected from the MDR-TB patients through the interview schedules, General Health Questionnaire (GHQ 12) with and Internalised Stigma of Mental Illness (ISMI) scale.

The Secondary Data

The secondary sources consisted of the research studies, magazines, journals, research articles, books and the reports from the WHO Annual Report, India TB report, RNTCP and State wise TB report.

The authors has also obtained information from the TB medical experts, DOTS plus site, Culture and DST Lab for TB and MDR-TB at ICMR National Institute for Research in Tuberculosis, Chennai.

Pre-Test

Pre-tests were done for the following tools:

1. General Interview Schedule incorporating, Demographic & Personal, Socioeconomic condition, TB treatment, Current MDR-TB treatment, Family support, and Institutional support factors.
2. Psychological Well-being Scale was used with Likert Scale scoring to study the Psychological Well-being of MDR-TB patients by the authors.
3. General Health Questionnaire with Likert scale was used by the authors to pre-test the health status to study the evidence of psychological distress among the MDR-TB patients.
4. Internalized Stigma of Mental Illness Scale (ISMI) was used to pretest the internalized stigma and its related mental illness among the MDR-TB patients.
5. The tools were administered among 37 MDR-TB patients and modified the pre-tested tool with appropriate corrections before the final data collection. To mention few modifications, open-ended questions were incorporated with the options wherever it was necessary, the "not applicable" option wherever it was relevant, income slabs option was modified by grouped with more appropriate options and questions.

Data Collection

The data were collected data from patients at Greater Chennai Corporation, Urban Primary Health Centres (UPHC), which are run under the National Tuberculosis Elimination Programme (NTEP), Tuberculosis Treatment Centre (TB Unit) and where patients used to go for treatment and follow up, as well as collecting data from patients, During the same period, the authors used the Qualitative Research technique to conduct a 5-focus group discussion (FGD).

Ethical Considerations

The study upheld respondents' ("MDR-TB patients") rights to voluntary participation, informed consent, and confidentiality. A consent form was included with the data collection instruments to solicit respondents' voluntary participation in the study. The purpose of the study, the sort of information required, the purpose for which it will be used, the rationale for selecting them as participants, and how they are expected to participate were all specified in the form. Additionally, it was stated that their participation in the study is completely voluntary and that they may quit at any time.

Data Analysis

The collected primary data were analysed using the Statistical Package for Social Sciences (SPSS) 20th version. The authors used the descriptive statistical methods frequency tables, mean, standard deviation and percentages to describe the profile of MDR-TB patients. To explain the relationship among the variables authors used the inferential statistical tests such as Pearson Correlation Coefficient.

Interview Schedule

This was the first part of the tool which consists of demographic & personal profiles, such as Age, Gender, Religion, Educational Qualification, Marital Status, Family Type, Number of Family members in the family etc. were used and collected data and the data were entered in MS Excel and analyzed using SPSS software. The authors tries to describe through a test such as and Pearson Correlation Coefficient is used for booking the relationship between variables and analysis whether any significant relationship exists among the various profiles.

Psychological Well-being Scale

This scale was used with Likert Scale scoring to book the Psychological Well-being of MDR-TB patients by the authors. Authorss have used the 42-item PWB Scale (Ryff & Keyes, 1995; Curhan *et al.*, 2014). Respondents rate how strongly they agree or disagree with 42 statements using a 7-point scale (1 = strongly agree; 7 = strongly disagree).

The PWB Scale has six subscales: Autonomy, Environmental Mastery, Personal Growth, Positive Relationship with Others (Purpose in Life and Self-acceptance. Data was Besides, the research book examines the psychosocial well-being of MDR tuberculosis patients in Chennai Corporation. As a result, the research book focuses on describing the psychosocial characteristics of MDR-TB patients, which serves as a descriptive research design entered in MS Excel and analysed using SPSS software for windows. For comparison between mean scores of groups, an independent t-test was used.

General Health Questionnaire (GHQ 12)

This scalewas used with the Likert Scale scoring to book the psychological distress among the MDR-TB patients by the authors. The scores on the scale 0, 1, 2, 3 from left to right are recorded; the Score range was from 0 to 36. Scores about 11–12 are typical which means. Besides, the research book examines the psychosocial well-being of MDR tuberculosis patients in Chennai Corporation.

As a result, the research book focuscs on describing the psychosocial characteristics of MDR-TB patients, which serves as a descriptive research design. A normal, Score above 15 is considered as Evidence of Distress and a Score above 20 suggests Severe Problems and Psychological distress. Data were entered in MS Excel and analyzed using SPSS software for windows. For comparison between mean scores of groups, an independent t-test was used. The mean scores for different domains were used in the analysis.

Internalised Sigma of Mental Illness (ISMI) Scale

ISMI which measures the Alienation, Stereotype (labelling) Endorsements, Discrimination Experiences and Stigma Resistance, the data was collected from the respondents.

For calculating the overall score on this scale, the authors followed the instruction guidelines as per scale to get the score. Score items of questions 24–28 was recorded to get the correct results (score 1->, 2->3, 3->4, 4->1). After this, the scores on the single items were summed and divided by the total number of questions (that is 28). Then the mean score was derived. The higher the mean score, the greater the evidence of self-stigma was considered as per the scale.

Definition of the Terms

The authors had operationally defined the terms and the variables and these operational definitions have the backing of conceptual definitions which are cited for reference.

Tuberculosis

Tuberculosis (TB) is a disease caused by bacteria that are spread from person to person through the air. TB usually affects the lungs, but it can also affect other parts of the body, such as the brain, the kidneys, or the spine. In most cases, TB is treatable and curable; however, people with TB can die if they do not get proper treatment. Sometimes drug-resistant TB occurs when bacteria become resistant to the drugs used to treat TB. This means that the drug can no longer kill the TB bacteria.

Multi Drug Resistant Tuberculosis (MDR-TB)

Multidrug-resistant TB (MDR-TB) is caused by TB a bacterium that is resistant to at least isoniazid and rifampicin, the two most potent TB drugs. Multidrug-resistant TB (MDR-TB) is TB that does not respond to at least isoniazid and rifampicin, the 2 most powerful anti-TB drugs.

Psychological Well-being

Psychological well-being refers to inter-and intra-individual levels of positive functioning that can include one's relatedness with others and self-referent attitudes that include one's sense of mastery and personal growth. Subjective well-being reflects dimensions of affect judgments of life satisfaction.

Limitations of the Study

In academic research, there are certain limitations. This is cross-sectional and not interventional and the instruments and scales used by the public at large. This research takes place in participants above the age of 18. This book thus does not demonstrate the psychosocial health of patients under the age of 18. This book was exclusively carried out in Chennai. These are some of the limitations of the research.

CHAPTER 6

Socio-Demographic Profile of MDR-TB Patients

Introduction

In the previous chapter, the methodological aspects of the research were discussed. In this chapter, the authors present the health profile of the MDR-TB patients in Chennai Greater Corporation. The data were generated from the respondents, processed and analyzed to answer the research questions in the book. Qualitative and quantitative data were integrated and interpreted to conclude.

To explain the relationship among the variable's authors used the inferential statistical tests such as chi-square and t-tests. The analysis of the collected data from 289 MDR-TB patients is presented as per the following in the sixth chapter of the book.

- Quantitative data was Analyzed using SPSS 20th version.
- Data was presented in the form of tables and charts
- Analysis such as descriptive statistics, regression was done.
- Qualitative data was analyzed using Dedoose (online website for qualitative data analysis) transcription, translations and thematic analysis.
- This data collected were presents the data in tables, diagrams and charts; narrates analyses and interpretations; and explicates the conclusions and the models developed in the book. This has been divided into 9 parts as follows;
    - **Demographic Profile:** Focuses on the Demographic and personal Profile of MDR-TB patients such as Age, Gender, Religion, Educational Status, Marital Status and Family type, Members in the family and discuss the testing of the hypothesis.
    - **Socio-Economic profile:** Describes the Socioeconomic profile of MDR-TB patients such as the Employment status of

MDR-TB patients, Employment Sector, Monthly income of the MDR-TB patients, Family Monthly income, Living House type of MDR-TB patients, Monthly House rent paid, patients having Public Distribution (PDS) of ration and financial assistance received from Govt. for taking treatment for MDR-TB.

- **TB and MDR and TB Treatment Profile:** which includes the duration of treatment, Problems faced by the MDR-TB patients. Amount of Money spend related to this disease by the MDR-TB patients, Money spends related to this disease by the MDR-TB patients and discusses the various tests used for testing the hypobook.
- **The Family Support Profile:** Includes the details of family support during this illness, feeling of isolation by the family members, sleeping pattern, taking food with family members and usage of separate glass and plate and also describes the testing of the hypobook.
- **Institutional Support Received by MDR-TB Patients:** This section covers information such as the distance to the government hospital, opinions on government hospital treatment, opinions on government hospital personnel service, and sources of daily DOTS therapy. The Revised National Tuberculosis Control Programme (RNTCP), (currently called as National Tuberculosis Elimination Programme (NTEP) Chennai Health District wise book describes the health facility in Greater Chennai Corporation and the Tuberculosis unit.
- **Psychological Well-being of MDR-TB Patients:** Describes to assess the evidence of psychological distress among them and examines the testing of the hypothesis.
- **General Health of MDR-TB Patients:** using the General Health Questionnaire (GHQ-12). Focuses on the general health of MDR-TB Patients.
- **Stigma and Discrimination of MDR-TB Patients:** Discrimination Experiences and Stigma Resistance and describes.

- **Quantitative Data Analysis:** The authors try to describe through a test such as and Pearson Correlation Coefficient is used for booking the relationship between variables and analysis whether any significant relationship exists among the various profiles. The chapter ends with a discussion on the conclusions and implications with regard to the Psychosocial Well-being of Multi-Drug Resistant Tuberculosis (MDR-TB) Patients.
- **Qualitative Data Analysis: The Focus Group Discussion (FGD):** Analysis of Qualitative Data: Focus Group Discussions (FGDs): Qualitative Interviews elucidates the difficulties encountered by MDR tuberculosis patients. Qualitative data were processed using Dedoose (an online platform for qualitative data analysis), which included transcription, translation, and thematic analysis.

Demographic Profile of The Respondents

This part focuses on the basic demographic and personal profile of MDR-TB patients. Under the demographic profile data regarding MDR Patients, Gender. Age, Religion, education, marital status and family details were analyzed. The data has collected from two hundred and eighty-nine (289) MDR-TB patients from 5 Health Districts in Chennai Chennai (North, East, West, South and Central) of Chennai Corporation, those who are diagnosed for MDR-TB and taking treatment under the National Tuberculosis Elimination programme (NTEP) formerly known as the Revised National Tuberculosis Programme (RNTCP).

Table 6.1: Gender Wise Distribution of MDR-TB Patients

S. No.	*Gender*	*Chennai Corporation Health Districts*					*Total*
		North Chennai	*East Chennai*	*Central Chennai*	*West Chennai*	*South Chennai*	
1.	Male	71(24.6)	5719.7)	40(13.8)	22(7.6)	20(6.9)	210(72.7)
2.	Female	18(6.2)	20(6.9)	19(6.6)	14(4.8)	8(2.8)	79(27.3)
Total		**89(30.8)**	**77(26.6)**	**59(20.4)**	**36(12.5)**	**28(9.7)**	**289(100)**

Table 6.1 shows the Gender and Health district-wise distribution of MDR-TB patients. The total number of Male MDR-TB patients

were 72.7 per cent. Among the Male MDR-TB patients, in North Chennai were (24.6%), East Chennai (19.7%), Central Chennai (13.8%), West Chennai (7.6%) and South Chennai 6.9 per cent.

The Female respondent constituted around 27.3 per cent, among them respondents from North Chennai (6.2%), East Chennai (6.9%), Central Chennai (6.6%), West Chennai(4.8%) and South Chennai 2.8 per cent of female MDR-TB patients. It is observed that the Male MDR-TB patients were higher (72.7%) when compared to the female MDR-TB patients (27.3%) in Chennai Corporation Health Districts.

Table 6.2: Age & Health District Wise Distribution of MDR-TB Patients

S. No.	*Age (in years)*	*Chennai Corporation Health Districts*					*Total*
		North Chennai	*East Chennai*	*Central Chennai*	*West Chennai*	*South Chennai*	
1.	18 to 30	16(5.5)	22(7.6)	17(5.9)	10(3.5)	6(2.1)	71(24.6)
2.	31 to 40	17(5.9)	14(4.8)	4(1.4)	4(1.4)	3(1.0)	42(14.5)
3.	41 to 50	22(7.6)	18(6.2)	14(4.8)	6(2.1)	5(1.7)	65(22.5)
4.	51 to 60	22(7.6)	18(6.2)	14(4.8)	13(4.5)	6(2.1)	73(25.3)
5.	60 and above	12(4.2)	5(1.7)	10(3.5)	3(1.0)	8(2.8)	38(13.1)
Total		**89(30.8)**	**77(26.6)**	**59(20.4)**	**36(12.5)**	**28(9.7)**	**289(100)**

*The figures in the parentheses denote the column percentage.

The above table 6.2 shows the age and health district-wise distribution of the respondents. The MDR-TB patients in the age group of 18 to 30 years were one fourth (24.6%) of the MDR-TB patients. Among this age group of patients were in North Chennai (5.5%), East Chennai (7.6%), Central Chennai (5.9%), West Chennai (3.5%) and South Chennai 2.1 per cent of the respondents. The MDR-TB patients in the age group of 31 to 40 years were (14.5%), Among this age group of patients were in North Chennai (5.9%), East Chennai (4.8%), Central Chennai and West Chennai equally 1.4 per cent and in South Chennai only one per cent. The MDR-TB patients in the age group of 41 to 50 years were more than one fifth (22.5%) of the respondents. Among this age group of patients, 7.6 per cent were in North Chennai, East Chennai (6.2%), Central

Chennai (4.8%), West Chennai(2.1%) and 1.7 per cent and South Chennai.

The MDR-TB patients in the age group above 60. years were (13.1%), Among above 60 years of MDR-TB patients in North Chennai were (4.2%), East Chennai (1.7%), Central Chennai (3.5%), one per cent 1 West Chennai and in South Chennai 2.8 per cent of the patients in this age group. When it is compared among the five districts in Chennai with the age group of the MDR-TB patients, it is found that the majority (30.8%) of the MDR-TB patients were from North Chennai when compared to other districts. Next to North Chennai in the East Chennai were (26.6%) and Central Chennai is had (20.4%) in all the age group.

Secondly, it is also observed that, overall, one-fourth of the MDR-TB patients in the age group between 18–30 (24.6%) and 51 to 60 (25.3%) higher were the number of MDR-TB patients in all three districts.

Thirdly it is observed that a lower number of MDR-TB cases were in West Chennai (12.5%) and South Chennai and had below 10 per cent which is lower in all the age groups when compared to the other 3 districts in Chennai.

Table 6.3: Religion Wise Distribution of MDR-TB Patient

S. No	*Religion*	*Chennai Corporation Health Districts*					*Total*
		North Chennai	*East Chennai*	*Central Chennai*	*West Chennai*	*South Chennai*	
1.	Hindu	86(29.8)	70 24.2)	51(17.6)	33(11.4)	25(8.7)	265(91.7)
2.	Muslim	0(0.0)	6(2.1)	6(2.1)	2(0.7)	2(0.7)	16(5.5)
3.	Christian	3(1.0)	1(0.3)	2(0.7)	1(0.3)	1(0.3)	8(2.8)
Total		**89(30.8)**	**77(26.6)**	**59(20.4)**	**36 12.5)**	**28(9.7)**	**289(100)**

The above Table 6.3 reveals the religion-wise distribution of MDR-TB patients among the 5-health district in Chennai. It is observed that 91.7 per cent of the MDR-TB patients were Hindus, among them in the five-Health Districts in Chennai. It is observed that Hindus were the higher number in North Chennai (29.8%) and East Chennai (24.5%). But in Central Chennai 17.6 per cent West

Chennai 11.4 and South Chennai 8.5 per cent were a lower number of MDR-TB patients.

The number of patients who belongs to the Muslim community was 5.5 per cent, among them, it is observed that there are no Muslim patients in North Chennai. East and Central Chennai had equally 2.1 per cent and West and South Chennai also equally 0.7 per cent of the MDR patients among the Muslim religion.

The MDR-TB patients from the Christian community were 2.8 per cent, among them was one per cent from North Chennai, from Central Chennai were (0.7%) only. It is observed that East, West and South Chennai was a negligible number (0.3%) belongs to Christian Religion.

Table 6.4: Educational Qualification of MDR-TB Patients

Sl. No.	*Educational Qualification*	*Chennai Corporation Health Districts*					*Total*
		North Chennai	*East Chennai*	*Central Chennai*	*West Chennai*	*South Chennai*	
1.	Illiterate	7(2.4)	4(1.4)	5(1.7)	1(0.3)	4(1.4)	21(7.3)
2.	Primary level	19(6.6)	16(5.5)	11(3.8)	7(2.4)	7(2.4)	60(20.8)
3.	High School	31(10.7)	20(6.9)	25(8.7)	9(3.1)	11(3.8.)	96(33.2)
4.	Higher Secondary	18(6.2)	17(5.9)	11(3.8)	10(3.5)	1(0.3)	57(19.7)
5.	Under graduation	9(3.1)	10(3.5)	4(1.4)	3(1.0)	3(1.0)	29(10.0)
6.	Postgraduation	3(1.0)	9(3.1)	1(0.3)	5(1.7)	0(0.0)	18(6.2)
7.	Others	2(0.7)	1(0.3)	2(0.7)	1(0.3)	2(0.7)	8(2.8)
	Total	**89(30.8)**	**77(26.6)**	**59(20.4)**	**36(12.5)**	**28(9.7)**	**289(100)**

Table 6.4 shows that the respondent's education according to health district-wise distribution. 7.3 per cent of the MDR-TB patients were illiterate in Chennai among them 0.7 per cent of them had low, (5.5%) of them had evidence of Moderate level of autonomy and one per cent of them and had a high level of autonomy. The patients who studied primary education were 20.8 per cent, among them, 7.3 per cent of them from North Chennai, (10.7%) per cent of them had evidence of Moderate level of autonomy and 2.8 per cent of them had a high level of autonomy.

The patients who completed High school were 33.2 per cent, among them 8.7 per cent of them had a low level of autonomy, 19.7 per cent of them had evidence of a Moderate level of autonomy and 4.8 per cent of them had a high level of autonomy.

The patients who completed the higher secondary were 19.7 per cent, among them 0.7 per cent of them had a low level of autonomy, (5.5%) of them had evidence of Moderate level of autonomy and 1.7 per cent of them and had a high level of autonomy.

The patients who studied up to under graduation were ten per cent, among them 1.7 per cent of them had a low level of autonomy, (6.9%) per cent of them had evidence of Moderate level of autonomy and 1.4 per cent of them had a high level of autonomy.

The patients who studied up to postgraduation were 6.2 per cent, among them (1.7%) of them had a low level of autonomy, 3.1 per cent of them had evidence of a Moderate level of autonomy and 1.4 per cent of them had a high level of autonomy.

The patients those who studied other qualification were 2.8 per cent, among them (1.7%) of them had evidence of Moderate level of autonomy and only one per cent of them had a high level of autonomy.

In this book it is observed that (33.2%) of the MDR-TB patients were studied High school and 20.8 per cent of the respondents have studied the primary level of education followed by Higher secondary (19.7%), Under graduation (10.0%), illiterate (7.3%), Postgraduate 6.2 and others include Certificate course and Diploma holders (2.8%) per cent of the educational status among MDR-TB patients.

Table 6.5: Marital Status of the MDR-TB Patients

S. No.	*Marital Status*	*Chennai Corporation Health Districts*					*Total*
		North Chennai	*East Chennai*	*Central Chennai*	*West Chennai*	*South Chennai*	
1.	Unmarried	15(5.2)	19(6.6)	13(4.5)	9(3.1)	4(1.4)	60(20.8)
2.	Married	64(22.1)	52(18.0)	39(13.5)	25(8.7)	20(6.9)	200(69.2)
3.	Separated	4(1.4)	3(1.0)	2(0.7)	2(0.7)	0(0.0)	11(3.8)
4.	Widow/er	6(2.1)	3(1.0)	5(1.7)	0(0.0)	4(1.4)	18(6.2)
Total		**89(30.8)**	**77(26.6)**	**59(20.4)**	**36(12.5)**	**28(9.7)**	**289(100)**

Table 6.5 shows the marital status of the MDR-TB patients. The patients who have unmarried 20.8 per cent, among them from East Chennai were (5.2%), East Chennai (6.6%), Central Chennai (4.5%), West Chennai (3.2%) and South Chennai (1.4%) respectively. The patients who were married (69.2%) per cent, among them from North Chennai were (22.1), East Chennai Eighteen per cent, Central Chennai (13.5%), West Chennai (8.7%) and South Chennai (6.9%) respectively.

The patients who were separated were 3.8 per cent, among them 1.4 per cent of them from North Chennai, one per cent from East Chennai, 0.7 per cent from Central Chennai & West Chennai. There are no separated MDR-TB patients from South Chennai the patients who were widows/widowers 6.2 per cent, among them (2.1%) of them from North Chennai, East Chennai one per cent, Central Chennai (1.7%) There is no widow/er from West Chennai and 6.2 per cent form South Chennai respectively.

Table 6.6: Family Type of MDR-TB Patients

S. No.	*Type of family*	*Chennai Corporation Health Districts*					*Total*
		North Chennai	*East Chennai*	*Central Chennai*	*West Chennai*	*South Chennai*	
1	Joint Family	9(3.1)	7(2.4)	8(2.8)	5(1.7)	4(1.4)	33(11.4)
2	Nuclear Family	73(25.3)	67(23.2)	47(16.3)	30(10.4)	23(8.0)	240(83.0)
3	Not Applicable	7(2.4)	3(1.0)	4(1.4)	1(0.3)	1(0.3)	16(5.5)
Total		**89(30.8)**	**77(26.6)**	**59(20.4)**	**36(12.5)**	**28(9.7)**	**289(100)**

Table 6.6 shows the type of family of MDR-TB patients in Chennai Corporation, The patients who were living in the joint family were (11.4%). From North Chennai (3.1%), East Chennai (2.4%), Central Chennai (16.3%), West Chennai (10.4%) and South Chennai eight per cent respectively.

The patients who were living in the nuclear family were eighty-three per cent, among them from North Chennai 25.3 per cent, East Chennai (23.2%) Central Chennai & West Chennai. There are no separated MDR-TB patients from South Chennai.

The patients who were living in either nuclear family or joint family which were not eligible were 5.5 per cent, among them from North Chennai were (2.4%), East Chennai one per cent, Central Chennai (1.4%), West Chennai & South Chennai were equally 0.3 per cent.

It is observed that the majority (83.0%) of the MDR-TB patients live in the nuclear family system. 11.4 per cent were living in a Joint family system and the remaining 5.5 per cent of them were not applicable in both categories were negligible.

Table 6.7: Number of Family Members Living in MDR-TB Patient's Family

S. No.	*Number of Family Members*	*Chennai Corporation Health Districts*					*Total*
		North Chennai	*East Chennai*	*Central Chennai*	*West Chennai*	*South Chennai*	
1.	One	4(1.4)	7(2.4)	3(1.0)	3(1.0)	1(0.3)	18(6.2)
2.	Two	34(11.8)	31(10.7)	17(5.9)	16(5.5)	13(4.5)	111(38.4)
3.	3 to 5	47(16.3)	33(11.4)	38(13.1)	15(5.2)	14(4.8)	147(50.9)
4.	Above 5	4(1.4)	6(2.1)	1(0.3)	2(0.7)	0(0.0)	13(4.5)
	Total	**89(30.8)**	**77(26.6)**	**59(20.4)**	**36(12.5)**	**28(9.7)**	**289(100)**

Table 6.7 brings about the number of persons living in the MDR-TB patient family. The patients who were living with one family member were 6.2 per cent, among them from North Chennai1.4 per cent, East Chennai (2.4%) Central Chennai & West Chennai were equally one per cent and South Chennai were (1,3%) respectively. The patients who were living with two members in the family were 38.4 per cent, among them from North Chennai 11.8 per cent, East Chennai (10.7%) Central Chennai (5.9%) West Chennai (5.5%) and from South Chennai were (4.5%) respectively.

The patients who were living with 3 to 5 members in the family were 50.9 per cent, among them from North Chennai 16.3 per cent, East Chennai (11.4%) Central Chennai (13.1%), West Chennai (5.2%) and from South Chennai were (4.8%) respectively. The patients who were living with above 5 members in the family were 4.5 per cent, among them from North Chennai 1.4 per cent, East

Chennai (2.1%) Central Chennai (0.3%) from South Chennai were (4.5%) respectively and there is no one from South Chennai.

The respondents who had three-five members in their family were 50.9 per cent and two members were 38.4 per cent followed by a single person (6.2%) and above 5 members were 4.5 per cent. It can be seen that the number of patients who had three to five members in their family was higher (50.9%) in MDR-TB patient's families.

CHAPTER 7

Socio-Economic Profile

This part highlights the Socioeconomic condition of the MDR-TB patients from Chennai, with regard to the employment status, monthly income, family income, living conditions, government entitlements and which were analysed by the authors. In health socioeconomic condition is viewed as the Persons of higher socioeconomic status have a range of resources that benefit health; they hold an advantage in warding off whatever particular threats to health exist at a given time. Therefore, as risk factors that stratify health are eliminated, socioeconomic health disparities remain.

Table 7.1: Employment Status of MDR-TB Patients

Sl. No.	*Employment Status*	*Chennai Corporation Health Districts*					*Total*
		North Chennai	*East Chennai*	*Central Chennai*	*West Chennai*	*South Chennai*	
1.	Employed	47(16.3)	29(10.0)	27(9.3)	13(4.5)	12(4.2)	128(44.3)
2.	Unemployed	31(10.7)	34(11.8)	18(6.2)	14(4.8)	13(4.5)	110(38.1)
4.	Student	7(2.4)	9(3.1)	8(2.8)	5(1.7)	1(0.3)	30(10.4)
5.	Housewife	4(1.4)	5(1.7)	6(2.1)	4(1.4)	2(0.7)	21(7.3)
Total		89(30.8)	77(26.6)	59(20.4)	36(12.5)	28(9.7)	289(100)

Table 7.1 shows the employment status of the MDR-TB patient in Chennai. Among the respondents 44.3 per cent was employed during their illness and of them from North Chennai 16.3 per cent, East Chennai ten per cent, Central Chennai (9.3%), West Chennai (4.5%) per cent and South Chennai were (4.2%) respectively. The patients who were unemployed during their illness were 38.1 per cent, among them from North Chennai (10.7) per cent, East Chennai (11.8%), Central Chennai (6.2%), West Chennai (4.8%) per cent and South Chennai were (4.5%) respectively. The patients those who were student were 10.4 per cent, among them from North Chennai

(2.4) per cent, East Chennai (3.1%), Central Chennai (2.8%), West Chennai (1.7%) per cent and South Chennai were (0.3%) respectively.

Among the MDR-TB patients, 7.3 per cent of them were housewife who was affected by MDR-TB. The house wife's who were affected by TB was high (2.1%) in Central Chennai followed by East Chennai 1.7 and 1.4 in North Chennai and West Chennai and South Chennai were (0.7%) which was low (1.6%).

It is observed that the majority (44.3%) of the respondents were employed and (38.1%) were unemployed. 10.4 per cent of the respondents were Students. 7.3 per cent of them were housewives during their illness. Among the respondent's majority of them (44.3%) of the MDR-TB patient were employed during the illness, among them (16.3%) belongs to north Chennai and ten per cent from east Chennai. It was observed that 38.1 per cent of the respondents were unemployed, among them 11.8 per cent in east Chennai and 10.7 per cent in North Chennai.

Table 7.2: Type of Employment of MDR-TB Patients

Sl. No.	*Type of Employment*	*Chennai Corporation Health Districts*					*Total*
		North Chennai	*East Chennai*	*Central Chennai*	*West Chennai*	*South Chennai*	
1.	Government	5(1.7)	4(1.4)	4(1.4)	3(1.0)	1(0.3)	17(5.9)
2.	Private	9(3.1)	4(1.4)	7(2.4)	3(1.0)	0(0.0)	23(8.0)
3.	Labour/daily wages	27(9.3)	17(5.9)	13(4.5)	7(2.4)	9(3.1)	73(25.3)
4.	Self Employed	6(2.1)	4(1.4)	3(1.0)	0(0.0)	2(0.7)	15(5.2)
5.	Not Applicable	42(14.5)	48(16.6)	32(11.1)	23(8.0)	16(5.5)	161(55.7)
Total		**89(30.8)**	**77(26.6)**	**59(20.4)**	**36(12.5)**	**28(9.7)**	**289(100)**

Table 7.2 shows the respondents type of employment. The respondents who worked in the government sector were 5.9 per cent, among them 1,7 per cent of them from North Chennai followed by East Chennai and Central Chennai were 1.4 per cent equally distributed and one per cent from West Chennai and (0.3%) from South Chennai which was very low per cent of respondent working in government sector during their illness.

The respondents who worked in the private sector were eight per cent, among them 3,1 per cent of them from North Chennai followed by East Chennai were (1.4%), Central Chennai was 2,4 one per cent from West Chennai and There are no private-sector employees from South Chennai. Among the MDR-TB patients, one fourth (25.3%) were working as a labour/daily wages, among them,9.3 per cent of them from North Chennai followed by East Chennai were (5.9%), Central Chennai was 4.5 per cent, from West Chennai 2.4 per cent and 3.1 per cent from South Chennai.

The patients who were working as self-employed were 5.2 per cent, among them from North Chennai were (2.1%) followed by (1.4%) East Chennai, Central Chennai one per cent, South Chennai. There is no self-employed from west Chennai. (0.7%) of respondents had a low level of alienation among this group.

More than half (55.7%) of the respondents were not eligible for any employment. In this category from East Chennai were higher (16.6) followed by North Chennai (14.5%), Central Chennai (11.1%), West Chennai eight per cent and 5;5 from South Chennai which was low in this category. It can be noticed that the MDR-TB patients from those who are not eligible for any employment almost they are unemployed were high, which means that if the breadwinner is sick the family will suffer from loss of income.

Table 7.3: Monthly Income of the MDR-TB Patients

S. No.	*Monthly Income*	*Chennai Corporation Health Districts*					*Total*
		North Chennai	*East Chennai*	*Central Chennai*	*West Chennai*	*South Chennai*	
1.	Up to 5000	22(7.6)	12(4.2)	11(3.8)	4(1.4)	5(1.7)	54(18.7)
2.	5001 to 10000	17(5.9)	10(3.5)	6(2.1)	5(1.7)	6(2.1)	44(15.2)
3.	Above 10000	8(2.8)	7(2.4)	9(3.1)	4(1.4)	1(0.3)	29(10.0)
4.	Not Applicable	42(14.5)	48(16.6)	33(11.4)	23(8.0)	16(5.5)	162(56.1)
Total		**89(30.8)**	77(26.6)	**59(20.4)**	**36(12.5)**	**28(9.7)**	**289(100)**

From the above table 7.3, it can be observed that 18.7 per cent of the MDR-TB patients were earning an income of Rs. upto 5000 per month. The monthly salary e of MDR-TB patients in a range between Rs. 5001 to Rs. 10, 000/- were 15.2 per cent. The MDR-TB patients who were drawing a monthly salary above Rs. 10, 000/- were 10 per cent.

More than half (56.1) of the patients did not process any monthly income or salary during the illness, among them, the majority (16.6%) of them were from East Chennai and followed by North Chennai were 14,5 per cent, Central Chennai (11.4%). West Chennai (8.0%) and South Chennai (5.5%) which was low.

Table 7.4: Total Family Monthly Income of the MDR-TB Patients

S. No.	*Family Monthly income*	*Chennai Corporation Health Districts*					*Total*
		North Chennai	*East Chennai*	*Central Chennai*	*West Chennai*	*South Chennai*	
1.	Below 5000	26(9.0)	6(2.1)	7(2.4)	7(2.4)	4(1.4)	50(17.3)
2.	5001 to 10000	21(7.3)	23(8.0)	20(6.9)	6(2.1)	8(2.8)	78(27.0)
3.	Above 10000	42(14.5)	48(16.6)	32(11.1)	23(8.0)	16(5.5)	161(55.7)
Total		**89(30.8)**	**77(26.6)**	**59(20.4)**	**36(12.5)**	**28(12.5)**	**289(100)**

Table 7.4 brings about the total family income of the MDR-TB patients. It can be observed that 17.3 per cent of the patient family income was below Rs. 5000/- per month, the patient's family which had a monthly income in the range of Rs. 5001 to 10000/- was twenty-seven per cent, It is observed that the patient's family which had an income of Rs. 10000/- and Above was 55.7 per cent.

Table 7.5: Total Monthly Income of MDR-TB Patients' Family

Sl. No.	*Education*	*Monthly Income of Patient's Family*			*Total*
		Up to 5000	*5001 to 10000*	*Above 10000*	
1.	Illiterate	2(0.7)	10(3.5)	9(3.1)	21(7.3)
2.	Primary level	14(4.8)	14(4.8)	32(11.1)	60(20.8)
3.	High School	13(4.5)	23(8.0)	60(20.8)	96(33.2)
4.	Higher Secondary	10(3.5)	20(6.9)	27(9.3)	57(19.7)
5.	Under graduation	5(1.7)	4(1.4)	20(6.9)	29(10.0)
6.	Post-graduation	1(0.3)	6(2.1)	11(3.8)	18(6.2)
7.	Other courses	5(1.7)	1(0.3)	2(0.7)	8(2.8)
Total		**50(17.3)**	**78(27.0)**	**161(55.7)**	**289(100)**

Table 7.5 shows that the respondent's family educational status according to their monthly income. The illiterate patients were 7.3 per cent, among them (0.7%) of them are earning up to Rs. 5000/- per month, 3,5% of them are earning Rs. 5001 to 10000 and 3.2 per cent of them earning Rs. 5000/- and above. The patients who studied primary education were 20.8 per cent, among them 4.8 per cent earning up to Rs. 5000/- and Rs. 5001 to 10000 and the remaining 11.1 per cent of them earning Rs. 5000/- and above per month.

The patients who completed High school were 33.2 per cent, among them (4.5%) per cent of them earning up to Rs. 5000/-, eight per cent of them earning Rs. 5001 to 10000 and the remaining 20.8 per cent of them earning Rs. 5000/- and above per month. The patients who completed the higher secondary were 19.7 per cent, among them 3.5 per cent of them the earning up to Rs. 5000/-, (6.9%) of them earning Rs. 5001 to 10000 and remaining 20.8 per cent of them earning Rs. 5000/- and above per month.

The patients who studied under graduation were ten per cent, among them 4.8 per cent of them earning up to Rs. 5000/- and 1.4 of them were earning Rs. 5001 to 10000 and remaining 11.1 per cent of them earning Rs. 5000/- and above per month. The patients who completed then Postgraduation were (6.2) per cent, among them 0.3 per cent of them earning up to Rs. 5000/-, (2.1%) of them earning Rs. 5001 to 10000 and remaining 20.8 per cent of them earning Rs. 5000/- and above per month. The patients who completed other educational status were (2.8) per cent, among them 1.7 per cent of them earning up to Rs. 5000/-, (0.3) of them earning Rs. 5001 to 10000 and remaining 0.7 per cent of them earning Rs. 5000/- and above per month. In this table, it is observed that more than half (55.7) of them earning Rs. above 10000 and one fourth (27.0) of them earning Rs 5001 to 10000. It is also observed that those who have studied up to High school were one fifth (20.8) of them were earning Rs. Above 10000/-.

Table 7.6 shows the earning members in the MDR-TB patient family. It can be noticed that around two-third (63%) of the respondents had single-member earnings in their families and among them, there were (19.7%) per cent in North Chennai, 17.3 per cent in East Chennai, 13.1 Percept in Central Chennai, 6.9 in West Chennai and 5. 9 in South Chennai.

Table 7.6: Earning Members in the MDR-TB Patients' Family

Sl. No.	*No of Earning Members*	*Chennai Corporation Health Districts*					*Total*
		North	*East*	*Central*	*West*	*South*	
1.	One	57(19.7)	50(17.3)	38(13.1)	20(6.9)	17(5.9)	182(63.0)
2.	Two	26(9.0)	24(8.3)	18(6.2)	10(3.5)	9(3.1)	87(30.1)
3.	3 to 5	3(1.0)	1(0.3)	2(0.7)	4(1.4)	1(0.3)	11(3.8)
4.	Above 5	1(0.3)	2(0.7)	0(0.0)	1(0.3)	0(0.0)	4(1.4)
5.	Not Applicable	2(1.4)	0(0.0)	1(0.3)	1(0.3)	1(0.3)	5(1.7)
Total		**89(30.8)**	**77(26.6)**	**59(20.4)**	**36(12.5)**	**28(9.7)**	**289(100)**

Table 7.7: House Type of the MDR-TB Patients

Sl. No.	*Type of house*	*Chennai Corporation Health Districts*					*Total*
		North	*East*	*Central*	*West*	*South*	
1.	Own House	20(6.9)	33(11.4)	29(10.0)	19(6.6)	10(3.5)	111(38.4)
2.	Rented	42(14.5)	25(8.7)	5(1.7)	6(2.1)	5(1.7)	83(28.7)
3.	Lease	14(4.8)	7(2.4)	9(3.1)	5(1.7)	4(1.4)	39(13.5)
4.	Not Applicable	13(4.5)	12(4.2)	16(5.5)	6(2.1)	9(3.1)	56(19.4)
Total		**89(30.8)**	**77(26.6)**	**59(20.4)**	**36(12.5)**	**28(9.7)**	**289(100)**

Table 7.7 shows the type of house in which MDR-TB patient lives. It is evident from the above table that the majority (38.4) of patients had their own house. The number of patients who lived in rented houses was 28.7 per cent. patients had their lease home were (13.5). The patients who did not pose any house or who shared that the housing type was not applicable were (19.4).

Table 7.8: Monthly House Rent Paid by MDR-TB Patient

S. No.	*House Rent*	*Chennai Corporation Health Districts*					*Total*
		North	*East*	*Central*	*West*	*South*	
1.	Below 2000	9(3.1)	2(0.7)	1(0.3)	2(0.7)	1(0.3)	15(5.2)
2.	2000 to 5000	14(4.8)	9(3.1)	1(0.3)	2(0.7)	2(0.7)	28(9.7)
3.	5001 to 10000	19(6.6)	15(5.2)	3(1.0)	1(0.3)	2(0.7)	40(13.8)
4.	>10000	34(11.8)	39(13.5)	38(13.1)	25(8.7)	14(4.8)	150(51.9)
	NA	13(4.5)	12(4.2)	16(5.5)	6(2.1)	9(3.1)	56(19.4)
Total		**89(30.8)**	**77(26.6)**	**59(20.4)**	**36(12.5)**	**28(9.7)**	**289(100)**

Table 7.8 reveals the monthly house rent paid by the MDR-TB patient. 5.2 per cent of the patients paid a monthly rent below Rs. 2000/- per month. It was observed that 9.7 per cent of the patients pay rent between Rs. 2001/- to 5000/- per month. The patients who paid monthly rent between Rs. 5001/- to 10,000/- were (13.8). A majority (51.9) of the MDR-TB patients paid Rs. 10000 above. 19.4 per cent did not pay any monthly house rent, it is observed that more than half (51.9%) of the MDR-TB patients have paid monthly house rent, among them from north Chennai 11.8 per cent, East Chennai 13.5 per cent, central Chennai 13.1 per cent, West Chennai 8.7 per cent and 4.8 per cent from South Chennai.

Table 7.9: MDR-TB Patients having Public Distribution System (PDS) Ration Card

Sl. No.	*Having Ration Card & Financial Assistance Received*	*Chennai Corporation Health Districts*					*Total*
		North	*East*	*Central*	*West*	*South*	
1.	Yes	60(20.8)	46(15.9)	40(13.8)	25(8.7)	18(6.2)	189(65.4)
	No	29(10.0)	31(10.7)	19(6.6)	11(3.8)	10(3.5)	100(34.6)
2.	Yes	64(22.1)	52(18.0)	34(11.8)	24(8.3)	16(5.5)	190(65.7)
	No	25(8.7)	25(8.7)	25(8.7)	12(4.2)	12(4.2)	99(34.3)
Total		**89(30.8)**	**77(26.6)**	**59(20.4)**	**36(12.5)**	**28(9.7)**	**289(100)**

As given in table 7.9 majority (65.4) of the MDR-TB patient's families have a Public Distribution Service (PDS) or a Ration Card for obtaining monthly food grains for family members from the State government. Among the patients who possessed ration cards, it is observed that 34.6 per cent of the MDR-TB patient family did not have PDS or Ration cards. The majority (65.7) of the MDR-TB patient's financial assistance was received from Govt. for taking treatment for MDR-TB. It is observed that 34.3 per cent of the MDR-TB patient did not receive financial assistance from Govt. for taking treatment for MDR-TB.

that they were age between 31 to 40 years were 14,5 per cent. Among them, less than one year of treatment was 6.6 per cent and 1 to 2 years was eight per cent.

Table 8.2: Age and Duration of the MDR TB Treatment

Sl. No.	*Age of the Patients*	*Duration of the MDR TB treatment*		*Total*
		Less than 1 year	*1 to 2 years*	
1.	18 to 30 years	22(7.6)	49(17.0)	71(24.6)
2.	31 to 40 years	19(6.6)	23(8.0)	42(14.5)
3.	41 to 50 years	33(11.4)	32(11.1)	65(22.5)
4.	51 to 60 years	30(10.4)	43(14.9)	73(25.3)
5.	60 years above	13(4.5)	25(8.7)	38(13.1)
Total		**117(40.5)**	**172(59.5)**	**289(100)**

The patients who shared that they were below the age between 41 to 50 years were 22.5 per cent. Among them, less than one year of treatment was 11.4 per cent and 1 to 2 years was 11.1 per cent. The patients who shared that they were age between 51 to 60 years were 25.3 per cent. Among them, less than one year of treatment was 10.4 per cent and 1 to 2 years was 14.9 per cent. The patients who shared that they were below the age between 60 years and above were 13.1 per cent. Among them, less than one year of treatment was 4.5 per cent and 1 to 2 years were 8.7 per cent.

It is observed that the age and duration of MDR TB treatment between 1 to 2 years were seventeen per cent belongs to the age group between 18 to 30 years followed by the age group between 51 to 60 were 14,9 per cent

The below table 8.3 shows the expenditure of money related to TB and other ailments of MDR TB patients during MDR TB treatment in Greater Chennai Corporation. Among the respondents' 21.1 per cent of the MDR TB patients had spent money on the diagnosis of TB and another ailment. 14.9 per cent had spent food for TB and another ailment, 17 per cent had spent money for food items during their MDR TB treatment. The majority (47.1) of the patients spent money on their travel during MDR TB treatment.

CHAPTER 8

Tuberculosis (TB) and Multi-Drug Tuberculosis (MDR TB) Treatment Profile

This part focuses on the TB treatment profiles which includes the duration of the treatment of MDR TB Patients, Treatment centre, Problems faced by the MDR TB patients, Amount of Money spent related to this disease by the MDR TB patients, Money spent related to this disease by the MDR TB patients for Diagnosis, to buy medicine and food.

Table 8.1: Duration of TB Illness of MDR TB Patient

S. No.	*Duration of TB Problem*	*Chennai Corporation Health Districts*					*Total*
		North Chennai	*East Chennai*	*Central Chennai*	*West Chennai*	*South Chennai*	
1.	Less than 1 year	44(15.2)	39(13.5)	12(4.2)	12(4.2)	10(4.2)	117(40.5)
2.	1 to 2 years	45(15.6)	38(13.1)	47(16.3)	24(8.3)	18(6.2)	172(59.5)
	Total	**89(30.8)**	**77(26.6)**	**59(20.4)**	**36(12.5)**	**28(9.7)**	**289(100)**

The above table 8.1 reveals that the duration of TB illness by the MDR TB patient. The patients who shared that they were unwell due to TB less than a year were 40.5 per cent, among them the patients who were unwell for one year to 2 years were more than half (59.5%) per cent.

The below table 8.2 reveals that the age and duration of MDR TB treatment have been taken by the respondents. The patients who shared that they were below the age between 18 to 30 years were 24.6 per cent. Among them, less than one year of treatment was 7.6 per cent and 1 to 2 years was seventeen per cent. The patients who shared

Table 8.3: Expenditure Made for TB/MDR TB Treatment

Sl. No.	*Money spend for*	*Chennai Corporation Health Districts*					*Total*
		North Chennai	*East Chennai*	*Central Chennai*	*West Chennai*	*South Chennai*	
1.	Diagnosis	17(5.9)	19(6.6)	12(4.2)	8(2.8)	5(1.7)	61(21.1)
2.	To buy medicine	9(3.1)	11(3.8)	12(4.2)	3(1.0)	8(2.8)	43(14.9)
3.	Food	31(10.7)	8(2.8)	4(1.4)	3(1.0)	3(1.0)	49(17.0)
4.	Travel	32(11.1)	39(13.5)	31(10.7)	22(7.6)	12(4.2)	136(47.1)
	Total	**89(30.8)**	77(26.6)	59(20.4)	**36(12.5)**	28(9.7)	**289(100)**

Table 8.4: Problem Faced by the MDR TB Patients

Sl. No.	*What Kind of Problem*	*Chennai Corporation Health Districts*					*Total*
		North Chennai	*East Chennai*	*Central Chennai*	*West Chennai*	*South Chennai*	
1.	Toxic Side effects	16(5.5)	7(2.4)	10(3.5)	5(1.7)	4(1.4)	42(14.5)
2.	Economical	31(10.7)	20(6.9)	10(3.5)	9(3.1)	11(3.8)	81(28.0)
3.	Social	12(4.2)	4(1.4)	8(2.8)	2(0.7)	1(0.3)	27(9.3)
4.	Others	30(10.4)	46(15.9)	31(10.7)	20(6.9)	12(4.2)	139(48.1)
Total		**89(30.8)**	77(26.6)	59(20.4)	**36(12.5)**	28(9.7)	**289(100)**

The above table 8.4 reveals those who have faced problems during the MDR TB treatment. Among the total respondent's 14.5 per cent of the MDR TB patients are faced Toxic side effects. 28 per cent of them faced the economic problem. 9.3 per cent of the patients have faced social problems. Among the total respondents (majority) 48.1 per cent did not face any problem during the MDR TB treatment

The below table 8.5 reveals that the relationship between the feeling during treatment of MDR TB patients. The patient group those who were better feeling during treatment were (41.5%) per cent, among them those who from North Chennai were (16.6%), East Chennai (9.7%) Central Chennai (6.9%), West Chennai (4.5%) and 3.8 per cent from south Chennai.

Table 8.5: MDR TB Patients Feeling During the Treatment

Sl No.	*Felling of the Patient During Treatment*	*Chennai Corporation Health Districts*					*Total*
		North Chennai	*East Chennai*	*Central Chennai*	*West Chennai*	*South Chennai*	
1.	Better	48(16.6)	28(9.7)	20(6.9)	13(4.5)	11(3.8)	120(41.5)
2.	Same	22(7.6)	33(11.4)	29(10.0)	11(3.8)	14(4.8)	109(37.7)
3.	Worsen	8(2.8)	14(4.8)	(0.0)	6(2.1)	3(1.0)	31(10.7)
4.	No Response	11(3.8)	2(0.7)	10(3.5)	6(2.1)	0(0.0)	29(10.0)
	Total	**89(30.8)**	**77(26.6)**	**59(20.4)**	**36(12.5)**	**28(9.7)**	**289(100)**

The patients who were the same feeling during treatment were (37.7%) per cent. The patient group who was the same feeling during treatment were ten per cent, among them those who from North Chennai, East Chennai (11.4%) Central Chennai (6.9%), West Chennai (3.8%) and 4.8 per cent from south Chennai. The patients who had to worsen feelings during treatment were (10.7), among them those who from North Chennai was (2.8%), East Chennai 4.8%), West Chennai (2.1%) and one per cent from south Chennai.

The patients who were not responding about the feeling during treatment were ten per cent, among them those who from North Chennai were (3.8%), East Chennai (0.7%), Central Chennai (3.5%) and West Chennai (2.1%). According to the above table, the relationship between the feeling during treatment of MDR TB patients is as follows: those who had a better feeling during treatment were (41.5 per cent) from North Chennai (16.6), while those who had a worse feeling during treatment were (9.7%) from East Chennai. A similar sentiment exists in East Chennai (11.4 per cent) and Central Chennai (ten per cent).

CHAPTER 9

Family Support Profile

This part includes the profile of family support to MDR TB patients during the treatment, which includes the details of family support during this illness, isolation by the family members, sleeping pattern, taking food with family members and usage of separate glass and plate. The family support to the MDR TB patients is analyzed in this section.

Table 9.1: Family Support Received by the Patients During Illness

Sl. No.	*Family Support*	*Chennai Corporation Health Districts*					*Total*
		North Chennai	*East Chennai*	*Central Chennai*	*West Chennai*	*South Chennai*	
1.	Yes	14(4.8)	36(12.5)	12(4.2)	6(2.1)	3(1.0)	71(24.6)
2.	No	75(26.0)	41(14.2)	47(16.3)	30(10.4)	25(8.7)	218(75.4)
Total		**89(75.4)**	**77(26.6)**	**59(20.4)**	**36(12.5)**	**28(9.7)**	**289(100)**

Table 9.1 reveals that the family support received by the patients during MDR TB treatment. 24.6 per cent of the patient's received family support during illness and treatment. Among the total respondents (4.8%) from North Chennai, (12.5%) East Chennai, (4.2%) Central Chennai, (2.1%) West Chennai and form South Chennai one per cent.

It can be observed that the majority of the respondents (75.4%) of the MDR TB patients have not received support from the family during their TB illness, among these patients twenty-six per cent of them were from North Chennai, 14.2 per cent of them were from East Chennai, 16.3 per cent West Chennai, 10.4 per cent East Chennai and 8.7 per cent of them were from South Chennai.

Table 9.2: Feeling of Isolation by the MDR TB Patients

Sl. No.	*Feeling Isolation*	*Chennai Corporation Health Districts*					*Total*
		North Chennai	*East Chennai*	*Central Chennai*	*West Chennai*	*South Chennai*	
1.	Yes	62(21.5)	57(19.7)	25(8.7)	17(5.9)	17(5.9)	178(61.6)
2.	No	27(9.3)	20(6.9)	34(11.8)	19(6.6)	11(3.8)	111(38.4)
	Total	**89(30.8)**	**77(26.6)**	**59(20.4)**	**36(12.5)**	**28(9.7)**	289(100)

The above Table 9.2 shows the district-wise distribution with the feeling of isolation by the MDR TB patients from their family members. In the above table (61.6%) per cent of the respondents shared that they were isolated by their family members due to MDR TB, among these patients 21.5 per cent of them were from North Chennai, (19.7%) per cent of them were from East Chennai, (8.7%) from Central Chennai, 5.9 per cent of them were from West Chennai and (5.9%) of them from South Chennai.

38.4 per cent of the respondents shared that they were not isolated by their family members, among these patients 9.3 per cent were from North Chennai, (26.6%) per cent of them were from East Chennai, (20.4%) from Central Chennai, 12.5 per cent of them were from West Chennai and (9.7%) of them from South Chennai.

It was observed that the majority 61.6 per cent of the respondents shared that they were isolated by their family members due to MDR TB. Some (38.4) of the respondents shared that they were not isolated by their family members

Table 9.3: Sleeping Pattern of MDR TB patients

Sl. No	*Sleep Pattern*	*Chennai Corporation Health Districts*					*Total*
		North Chennai	*East Chennai*	*Central Chennai*	*West Chennai*	*South Chennai*	
1.	With my family members	29(10.0)	37(12.8)	22(7.6)	8(2.8)	15(5.2)	111(38.4)
2.	sleep separately	60(20.8)	40(13.8)	37(12.8)	28(9.7)	13(4.5)	178(61.6)
	Total	**89(30.8)**	77(26.6)	**59(20.4)**	**36(12.5)**	**28(9.7)**	**289(100)**

The above Table 9.3 shows the state-wise distribution of MDR TB patients' sleeping patterns. It can be observed that 38.4 per cent of MDR TB patients slept with family members, that 10 per cent of patients were from North Chennai, that the highest (12.8 per cent) of patients were from East Chennai, that 7.6 per cent of patients were from central Chennai, that (2.8 per cent) of patients were from South Chennai, and that 5.2 per cent of patients were from South Chennai.

The majority (61.6%) of respondents reported sleeping separately from family members, with the majority (20.8%) from East Chennai, 13.8% from Central Chennai, 9.7% from West Chennai, and 4.5% from South Chennai. Because of MDR TB, the great majority of responders (61.6 per cent) reported sleeping separately from their family members. Several respondents (38.4) stated that MDR TB patients slept with family members when ill with MDR TB.

Table 9.4: Taking Daily Food with Family Members

Sl	*Food with Family*	*Chennai Corporation Health Districts*					*Total*
		North Chennai	*East Chennai*	*Central Chennai*	*West Chennai*	*South Chennai*	
1.	Yes	43(14.9)	36(12.5)	31(10.7)	18(6.2)	7(2.4)	135(46.7)
2.	No	46(15.9)	41(14.2)	28(9.7)	18(6.2)	21(7.3)	154(53.3)
	Total	**89(30.8)**	77(26.6	**59(20.4)**	**36(12.5)**	**28(9.7)**	**289(100)**

Table 9.4 shows whether the patient takes the daily food along with the family members or the patient is being provided food separately due to TB illness. It is noticed that 46.7 per cent of the MDR TB patients takes the daily food along with their family members, among these patients 14.9 per cent of them were from North Chennai, (12.5%) from East Chennai, 10.7 per cent of the patients were from Central Chennai, 6.2 per cent of the patients were from West Chennai and 2.4 per cent form south Chennai.

53.3 per cent of the respondents shared that they were being provided food separately due to TB illness, among them (15.9%) patients were from North Chennai, 14.2 per cent from East Chennai, (9.7%) from Central Chennai, (6.2%) from West Chennai and 7.3 per cent of the patients belonged to South Chennai. It is noticed that 46.7 per cent of the MDR TB patients take the daily food along with their family members and 53.31 per cent of the respondents shared that they were being provided food separately due to TB illness.

Table 9.5: Provision of the Place of Access at Home

Sl. No.	*Separate Plate and Glass Provided*	*Chennai Corporation Health Districts*					*Total*
		North Chennai	*East Chennai*	*Central Chennai*	*West Chennai*	*South Chennai*	
1.	Yes	31(10.7)	31(10.7)	29(10.0)	16(5.5)	12(4.2)	119(41.2)
2.	No	58(20.1)	46(15.9)	30(10.4)	20(6.9)	16(5.5)	170(58.8)
	Total	**89(30.8)**	**77(26.6)**	**59(20.4)**	**36(12.5)**	**28(9.7)**	**289(100)**

Table 9.5 shows whether the patients were provided separate glasses and plates to take their food at home by their family members due to TB illness.

It was observed that 41.2 per cent of the MDR TB patients were using separate glass and plates to take their food at home provided by their family members due to this TB illness. Among these patients, 10.7 per cent is equally from North Chennai and East Chennai, Ten per cent from central Chennai, 5.5 per cent from West Chennai and 4.2 per cent from south Chennai.

A majority (58.8) of the respondents were not separate the Glass & Plate for taking food by their family members. It was observed that (41.2%) per cent of the MDR TB patients were using spate glass and plates to take their food at home provided by their family members due to this TB illness.

CHAPTER 10

Institutional Support Received by MDR-TB Patients

In this section, the institutional support for MDR-TB patients is being analyzed. The profile of the institutional support profile includes the referral person to the government hospital, distance to reach the government hospital, opinion on government hospital treatment, opinion on government hospital staff service and sources of taking MDR-TB treatment are being analyzed through this profile.

Table 10.1: Distance to Reach Govt. Health Facility from Patient's Residence

Sl. No	*Distance from Home*	*Chennai Corporation Health Districts*					*Total*
		North Chennai	*East Chennai*	*Central Chennai*	*West Chennai*	*South Chennai*	
1.	Less than 5 KM	34(11.8)	33(11.4)	30(10.4)	17(5.9)	21(7.3)	135(46.7)
2.	Above 5 KM	55(19.0)	44(15.2)	29(10.0)	19(6.6)	7(2.4)	154(53.3)
	Total	**89(30.8)**	**77(26.6)**	**59(20.4)**	**36(12.5)**	**28(9.7)**	**289(100)**

The above table provides information about the distance to the nearest Government health facility or Government hospital for TB treatment. Among the total respondents, 46.7 per cent of them shared that the Government health facility or Government hospital was in reach within less than 5km, among these patients 11.8 per cent of them were from North Chennai, patients from East Chennai were (11.4), 10.4 per cent of the patients were from Central Chennai, West Chennai (5.9) and (7.3) from South Chennai.

It was observed that more than half (53.3) of the MDR-TB patients shared that the Government health facility was in reach between above 5 km, among these patients 19.0 per cent of them were from North Chennai, patients from East Chennai were (15.2), Ten per cent of the patients were from Central Chennai, West Chennai (6.6) and (2.4) from South Chennai. A majority (53.3) of the MDR-TB patients shared that the Government health facility was in reach between 2 to 5 km. It was observed that more than half (53.3%) of the MDR-TB patients shared that the Government health facility was in reach between above 5 km. Among the total respondent's 46.7 per cent of them shared that the Government health facility or Government hospital to in reach within less than 5km.

Table 10.2: Opinion on Treatment Facility at Government Hospital

Sl. No.	*Opinion on Treatment Facility*	*Chennai Corporation Health Districts*					*Total*
		North Chennai	*East Chennai*	*Central Chennai*	*West Chennai*	*South Chennai*	
1.	Good	43(14.9)	40(13.8)	27(9.3)	14(4.8)	15(5.2)	139(48.1)
2.	Satisfactory	46(15.9)	37(12.8)	32(11.1)	22(7.6)	13(4.5)	150(51.9)
	Total	**89(30.8)**	**77(26.6)**	**59(20.4)**	**36(12.5)**	**28(9.7)**	**289(100)**

Table 10.2 shows the opinion of the MDR-TB patients on the Government facility or Government hospital facility in five districts in Chennai. Among the total respondent's (48.1) shared that the service provided at the Government health facility was Good according to them, among them they expressed their opinion was good were (14.9) from North Chennai, (13.8) from East Chennai, Central Chennai 9.3 per cent, West Chennai (4.8) and South Chennai were 5.2 per cent.

The majority of the patients who shared that the Government health facility service was Satisfactory were 51.9 per cent, among them 15.9 per cent of them were f (12.8) from North Chennai, (12.8) from East Chennai, Central Chennai 11.1 per cent, West Chennai (7.6) and South Chennai were 4.5 per cent. The respondents not shared that they can't say any opinion about the government health facility and its services.

Table 10.3: Opinion on Government Hospital Staff Service

S. No.	*Opinion on Government Hospital Staff Service*	*Chennai Corporation Health Districts*					*Total*
		North Chennai	*East Chennai*	*Central Chennai*	*West Chennai*	*South Chennai*	
1.	Good	49(17.0)	40(13.8)	41(14.2)	22(7.6)	16(5.5)	168(58.1)
2.	Satisfactory	40(13.8)	37(12.8)	18(6.2)	14(4.8)	12(4.2)	121(41.9)
	Total	**89(30.8)**	77(26.6)	**59(20.4)**	**36(12.5)**	**28(9.7)**	**289(100)**

Table 10.3 shows the opinion of the MDR-TB patients on the Government health staff service at the hospital during their treatment in five districts. The majority (58.1) of the patients shared that the Government Health Staff behaviour and their service was good at the Government health facility, among them they expressed their opinion was good were (17) from North Chennai, East Chennai (13.8). Central Chennai 14.2 per cent, West Chennai (7.6) and South Chennai was 5.5 per cent.

The patients who shared that the Government Health Staff behaviour and their service as satisfactory was 41.9 per cent, among them majority (13.8) were from North Chennai, 12.8 per cent of them were from East Chennai 6.2 per cent of the patients were from Central Chennai, West Chennai 4.8 and South Chennai 4.2 per cent. The patients who not shared that they can't Say any opinion about the Government health staff service at the hospital.

It was observed that more than half (58.1) of the MDR-TB patients p shared that the Government Health Staff behaviour and their service was good at the Government health facility. The patients who shared that the Government Health Staff behaviour and their service as satisfactory were 41.9 per cent.

CHAPTER 11

Psychosocial Well-being (PWB) of MDR-TB Patients

This part includes the Psychological Well-being (PWB) of MDR-TB patients, The PWB Scale has six subscales: Autonomy (e.g., "I have confidence in my opinions, even if they are contrary to the consensus"); Environmental Mastery (e.g., "In general, I feel I am in charge of the situation in which I live"); Personal Growth (e.g., "I think it is important to have new experiences that challenge how you think about yourself and the world"); Positive Relationship With Others (e.g., "People would describe me as a giving person, willing to share my time with others"); Purpose in Life (e.g., "Some people wander through life, but I am not one of them"); and Self-acceptance (e.g., "When I look at the story of my life, I am pleased with how things have turned out").

The authors analyzed demographic and other variables with six subscales, which includes the details of Level of Autonomy, Level of Environmental Mastery, Level of Personal growth, level of a positive relationship, level of Purpose of life, Level of Self-Acceptance, level of psychological well-being, psychological well-being well-being of MDR-TB patients is analyzed in this section

Table 11.1: Level of Psychological Well-being

Sl. No.	*Level of Psychological Well-being*	*Frequency*	*Percent*
1.	Low	19	6.6
2.	Moderate	167	57.8
3.	High	103	35.6
	Total	**289**	**100**

The Level of Psychological Well-being (PWB) is shown in Table 11.1. PWB levels were observed in 6.6 per cent of MDR-TB patients.

A moderate level of PWB strikes 57.8% of patients, whereas a high level of PWB affects 35.5 per cent. The majority of MDR-TB patients have a Moderate level of psychological well-being, according to data.

Table 11.2: Sex and Level of Psychological Well-being

S. No.	*Sex*	*Level of Psychological Well-being*			*Total*
		Low	*Moderate*	*High*	
1.	Male	12(63.2)(4.2)	117(70.1)(40.5)	81(78.6)(28.0)	210(72.7)
2.	Female	7(36.8)(2.4)	50(29.9)(17.3)	22(21.4)(7.6)	79(27.3)
Total		**19(6.6)**	**167(57.8)**	**103(35.6)**	**289(100.0)**

Table 11.2 shows the gender and level of psychological well-being of MDR-TB patients. 4.2% of the 72.7 per cent of male respondents reported a low level of psychological well-being. However, 40.5 per cent of the patients had evidence of a moderate level of psychological well-being, whereas 28 per cent of the patients had evidence of a high level of psychological well-being.

Of the female respondents, 27.3 per cent have a poor level of psychological well-being, 2.4 per cent have a low level of psychological well-being, 17.3 per cent have a moderate level of psychological well-being, and 7.6 per cent have a high level of psychological well-being.

The majority of respondents (72.7%) were male, and there was evidence of a moderate level of psychological well-being, with almost half (40.5%) indicating a level of psychological well-being. When compared to females, there is evidence of moderate psychological well-being among 27.3 per cent of them (17.3 per cent).

Table 11.3: Age and Level of Psychological Well-being

Sl. No.	*Age of the Patients*	*Level of Psychological Well-being*			*Total*
		Low	*Moderate*	*High*	
1.	18 to 30 years	7(36.8)(2.4)	44(26.3)(15.2)	20(19.4)(6.9)	71(24.6)
2.	31 to 40 years	2(10.5)(0.7)	22(13.2)(7.6)	18(17.5)(6.2)	42(14.5)
3.	41 to 50 years	2(10.5)(0.7)	34(20.4)(11.8)	29(28.2)(10.0)	65(22.5)
4.	51 to 60 years	6(31.6)(2.1)	44(26.3)(15.2)	23(22.3)(8.0)	73(25.3)
5.	Above 60 years	2(10.5)(0.7)	23(13.8)(8.0)	13(12.6)(4.5)	38(13.1)
Total		**19(6.6)**	**167(57.8)**	**103(35.6)**	**289(100)**

Table 11.3 shows the age and level of psychological well-being of MDR-TB patients according to their age. The patients who were age between 18 to 30 years were 24.6 per cent, among them 2.4 per cent of them had a level of psychological well-being. 15.2 per cent of them had a moderate level of psychological well-being and 6.9 per cent of them had a high level of psychological well-being. The patients who were age between 31 to 40 years were 14.5 per cent, among them 0.7 per cent of them had a low level of psychological well-being, 7.6 per cent of them had evidence of a moderate level of psychological well-being and (6.2%) of them had a high level of psychological well-being. The patients who were age between 41 to 50 years were 22.5 per cent, among them 0.7 per cent of them had a low level of psychological well-being, (11.8%) per cent of them had a moderate level of self-acceptance and ten per cent of them had a high level of psychological well-being.

The patients who were age between 51 to 60 years were 25.3 per cent, among them 2.1 per cent of them had a low level of psychological well-being, 15.2 per cent of them had a moderate level of psychological well-being and eight per cent of them had a high level of psychological well-being.

The patients who were age between above 60 years were 13.1 per cent, among them 0.7 per cent of them had a low level of psychological well-being, eight per cent of them had a moderate level of psychological well-being and 4.5 per cent of them had a high level of psychological well-being. It is observed that the patients who were age between 18 to 30 years were (24.6) and among them (15.2) per cent of them had a moderate level of psychological well-being and the

Table 11.4: Religion and Level of Psychological Well-being

Sl. No.	*The Religion of the Patients*	*Level of Psychological Well-being*			*Total*
		Low	*Moderate*	*High*	
1.	Hindu	18(94.7)(6.2)	153(91.6)(52.9)	94(91.3)(32.5)	265(91.7)
2.	Muslim	1(5.3)(0.3)	9(5.4)(3.1)	6(5.8)(2.1)	16(5.5)
3.	Christian	0(0.0)(0.0)	5(3.0)(1.7)	3(2.9)(1.0)	8(2.8)
Total		**19(6.6)**	**167(57.8)**	**103(35.6)**	**289(100)**

patients who were age between 51 to 60 years were (25.3%) and among them (15.2) per cent of them had Moderate level of psychological well-being.

Table 11.4 shows the religion and level of psychological well-being of MDR-TB patients according to their religion. The patients who belong to Hindu were (91.7%) per cent. Among them, (6.2%) had a low level of psychological well-being. Evidence of a moderate level of psychological well-being was noticed among 52.9 per cent and (32.5) per cent of them had a high level of psychological well-being. The patients who belong to the Muslim religion were (5.5) per cent. Among them, 0.3 per cent had low psychological well-being, and 3.1 per cent had evidence of a moderate level of psychological well-being. (2.1%) had a high level of psychological well-being.

The patients who belong to Christian were 2.8 per cent. Among them, there was no low level of psychological well-being. 1.7 per cent of them had a moderate level of psychological well-being and one per cent of them had a high level of psychological well-being.

Table 11.5: Education and Level of Psychological Well-being

Sl. No.	*Education*	*Level of Psychological well-being*			*Total*
		Low	*Moderate*	*High*	
1.	Illiterate	0(0.0)(0.0)	13(7.8)(4.5)	8(7.8)(2.8)	21(7.3)
2.	Primary level	4(21.1)(1.4)	30(18.0)(10.4)	26(25.2)(9.0)	60(20.8)
3.	High School	8(42.1)(2.8)	51(30.5)(17.6)	37(35.9)(12.8)	96(33.2)
4.	Higher Secondary	3(15.8)(1.0)	38(22.8)(13.1)	16(15.5)(5.5)	57(19.7)
5.	Under graduation	3(15.8)(1.0)	21(12.6)(7.3)	5(4.9)(1.7)	29(10.0)
6.	Post-graduation	1(5.3)(0.3)	11(6.6)(3.8)	6(5.8)(2.1)	18(6.2)
7.	Others	0(0.0)(0.0)	3(1.8)(1.0)	5(4.9)(1.7)	8(2.8)
Total		**19(6.6)**	**167(57.8)**	**103(35.6)**	**289(100)**

Table 11.5 shows the education and the level of psychological well-being of MDR-TB patients according to their educational qualifications. 7.3 per cent of the MDR-TB patients were illiterate. Among them, there was no low level of psychological well-being (4.5%) of them had evidence of a moderate level of psychological well-being and 2.8 per cent of them had a high level of psychological well-

being. The patients who were primary educational qualification were 20.8 per cent, among them 1.4 per cent of them had a low level of psychological well-being, (10.4%) per cent of them had evidence of a moderate level of psychological well-being and nine per cent of them had a high level of psychological well-being.

The patients who completed High school were 33.2 per cent, among them 2.8 per cent of them had a low level of psychological well-being, 17.6 per cent of them had evidence of a moderate level of psychological well-being and 12.8 per cent of them had a high level of 19.7 per cent of the MDR-TB patients were completed higher secondary, among them one per cent of them had a low level of psychological well-being, (13.1%) of them had evidence of a moderate level of psychological well-being and 5.5 per cent of them and had the level of psychological well-being.

The patients who studied up to under graduation were ten per cent, among them one per cent of them had a low level of psychological well-being 7.3 per cent and (1.7%) of them had evidence of a moderate level of psychological well-being and one per cent of them and had a high level of psychological well-being. The patients who studied up to postgraduation were 6.2 per cent, among them 0.3 per cent of them had a low level of psychological well-being, 3.8 per cent of them had evidence of a moderate level of psychological well-being and 2.1 per cent of the high level of psychological well-being.

The patients those who studied other qualification were 2.8 per cent, among them there is no evidence of the low level of psychological well-being. One per cent of them had a moderate level of psychological

Table 11.6: Marital Status and Level of Psychological Well-being

Sl. No.	*Marital Status*	*Level of Psychological Well-being*			*Total*
		Low	*Moderate*	*High*	
1.	Unmarried	7(36.8)(2.4)	35(21.0)(12.1)	18(17.5)(6.2)	60(20.8)
2.	Married	10(52.6)(3.5)	115(68.9)(39.8)	75(72.8)(26.0)	200(69.2)
3.	Separated	2(10.5)(0.7)	6(3.6)(2.1)	3(2.9)(1.0)	11(3.8)
4.	Widow/er	0(0.0)(0.0)	11(6.6)(3.8)	7(6.8)(2.4)	18(6.2)
Total		**19(6.6)**	**167(57.8)**	**103(5.6)**	**289(100)**

well-being and 1.7 per cent of them had a high level of psychological well-being. It is observed that those who have studied up to High school were 33.2 per cent among them nearly one fifth (17.6%) of them having evidence of a moderate level of psychological well-being.

Table 11.6 shows that the Marital Status and the psychological well-being of MDR-TB patients according to their Marital Status. Unmarried MDR-TB patients were 20.8 per cent, among them 2.4 per cent of them had a low level of psychological well-being, 12.1 per cent of them had evidence of Moderate psychological well-being and 6.2 per cent of them and had a high level of psychological well-being.

Of the patients who were married 69.2 per cent, among them 3.5 per cent of them had a low level of psychological well-being, (39.8%) per cent of them had evidence of a moderate psychological well-being and twenty-six per cent of them had a high level of psychological well-being.

It is observed that the majority 69.2 per cent of the respondents were married and among the married nearly half (45.7%) of them had evidence of a Moderate level of psychological well-being. The patients who were separated were 3.8 per cent, among them 0.7 per cent of them had low levels of psychological well-being, 2.1 per cent of them had evidence of Moderate psychological well-being and one per cent of them had a high level of psychological well-being.

The patients who were widows/er were 6.2 per cent, among them there is no low level of psychological well-being, 3.8 per cent of them had evidence of a moderate level of psychological well-being and 2.4 per cent of them had high psychological well-being among the widow/er participants.

Table 11.7: Type of Family and Level of Psychological Well-being

Sl. No.	*Type of family*	*Level of Psychological Well-being*			*Total*
		Low	*Moderate*	*High*	
	Joint Family	2(10.5)(0.7)	20(12.0)(6.9)	11(10.7)(3.8)	33(11.4)
2	Nuclear Family	16(84.2)(5.5)	137(82.0)(47.4)	87(84.5)(30.1)	240(83.0)
4	Not Applicable	1(5.3)(0.3)	10(6.0)(3.5)	5(4.9)(1.7)	16(5.5)
Total		**19(6.6)**	**167(57.8)**	**103(35.6)**	**289(100)**

It is observed that the patients who were married were 69.2 per cent and among this group majority (39.8%) of them had evidence of a moderate psychological well-being whereas the unmarried patients were (20.8%), among them (12.1%) per cent of them had a moderate level of psychological well-being.

Table 11.7 shows that the type of family and psychological well-being according to their type of family. The patients who were living in the joint family were 11.4 per cent, among them 0.7 per cent of them had a low level of psychological well-being, 6.9 per cent of them had evidence of a moderate level of psychological well-being and 3.8 per cent of them had a high level of psychological well-being. The patients who were living in the nuclear family were 83 per cent, among them 5.5 per cent of them had a low level of psychological well-being, 47.4 per cent of them had evidence of Moderate psychological well-being and 30.1 per cent of them had a high level of psychological well-being.

The remaining 5.5 per cent of them living with friends and hostel etc which was not applicable, among them 0.3 per cent of them had a low level of psychological well-being, 3.5 per cent of them had a moderate psychological well-being and 1.7 per cent of them had a high level of psychological well-being.

It is observed from the above table the type of family and psychological well-being of the MDR-TB patient's the majority 83% of them living in the nuclear family, among them nearly half (47.4%) of them had evidence of Moderate level of psychological well-being, when compared to the joint family were 11.4 per cent, among them the is evidence of Moderate psychological well-being had only 8 per cent, this shows that the joint family had the family support in connection with a positive relationship.

Table 11.8 shows the number of family members living with MDR-TB patients as well as their psychological well-being. There was 6.2 per cent of patients who lived with one family member, with 0.3 per cent having psychological well-being 3.8 per cent having evidence of a moderate degree of psychological well-being and 2.1 per cent having a high level of psychological well-being). The patients who lived with two family members accounted for 38.4 per cent of the total, with 2.8 per cent of them showing a level of psychological well-being, 24.4 per cent showing a moderate level of psychological well-being, and 15.2 per cent showing a high level of psychological well-being.

Table 11.8: Number of Family Members and Level of Psychological Well-being

Sl. No.	*Number of Family Members*	*Level of Psychological Well-being*			*Total*
		Low	*Moderate*	*High*	
1.	One	1(5.3)(0.3)	11(6.6)(3.8)	6(5.8)(2.1)	18(6.2)
2.	Two	8(42.1)(2.8)	59(35.3)(20.4)	44(42.7)(15.2)	111(38.4)
3.	3 to 5	8(42.1)(2.8)	88(52.7)(30.4)	51(49.5)(17.6)	147(50.9)
4.	Above 5	2(10.5)(0.7)	9(5.4)(3.1)	2(1.9)(0.7)	13(4.5)
Total		**19(6.6)**	**167(57.8)**	**103(35.6)**	**289(100)**

Patients who lived with 3 to 5 family members composed 50.9 per cent of the total, with 2.8 per cent having a low level of psychological well-being, 30.4 per cent having a moderate level of psychological well-being, and 17.6 per cent having a high level of psychological well-being.

It is observed that from the above table half of the MDR-TB patients (50.9%) were living with 3 to 5 number family members, among them, there is evidence of a Moderate level of psychological well-being of 30.4 per cent in the psychological well-being of MDR-TB patients

Table 11.9: Employment Status and Level of Psychological Well-being

Sl. No.	*Employment Status*	*Level of Psychological Well-being*			*Total*
		Low	*Moderate*	*High*	
1.	Employed	7(36.8)(2.4)	75(44.9)(26.0)	46(44.7)(15.9)	128(44.3)
2.	Unemployed	8(42.1)(2.8)	64(38.3)(22.1)	38(36.9)(13.1)	110(38.1)
3.	Student	4(21.1)(1.4)	15(9.0)(5.2)	11(10.7)(3.8)	30(10.4)
4.	Housewife	0(0.0)(0.0)	13(7.8)(4.5)	8(7.8)(2.8)	21(7.3)
Total		**19(6.6)**	**167(57.8)**	**103(35.6)**	**289(100)**

Table 11.9 shows that the employment status and level of psychological well-being of MDR-TB patients according to their

workplace. The patients who were employed were 44.3 per cent, among them 2.4 per cent of them had a low level of psychological well-being twenty-six per cent of them had evidence of a moderate level of psychological well-being and 15.9 per cent of them had a high level of psychological well-being. The unemployed patients were 38.1 per cent, among them 2.8 per cent of them had a low level of psychological well-being, 22.1 per cent of them had evidence of a moderate level of psychological well-being and 13.1 per cent of them had a high level of psychological well-being.

The patients those who were student were 10.4 per cent, among them 1.4 per cent of them had a low level of psychological well-being, 5.2 per cent of them had evidence of the moderate level of Psychological well-being and (3.8%) of them had a high level of psychological well-being.

The patients those who were housewife were 7.3 per cent, among them here is no low level of psychological well-being, (4.5%) of them had evidence of Moderate level of psychological well-being and 2.8 per cent of them had a high level of psychological well-being. According to the data as shown, MDR-TB patients who were employed (44.3 per cent) and unemployed (26.6 per cent) both had evidence of a moderate level of psychological well-being.

Table 11.10: Type of Employment and Level of Psychological Well-being

Sl. No.	*Employment Sector*	*Level of Psychological Well-being*			*Total*
		Low	*Moderate*	*High*	
1.	Government	0(0.0)(0.0)	16(9.6)(5.5)	1(1.0)(0.3)	17(5.9)
2.	Private	1(5.3)(0.3)	18(10.8)(6.2)	4(3.9(1.4)	23(8.0)
3.	Labour/daily wages	5(26.3)(1.7)	33(19.8)(11.4)	35(34.0)(12.1)	73(25.3)
4.	Self Employed	1(5.3)(0.3)	8(4.8)(2.8)	6(5.8)(2.1)	15(5.2)
5.	Not Applicable	12(63.2)(4.2)	92(55.1)(31.8)	57(55.3)(19.7)	161(55.7)
Total		**19(6.6)**	**167(57.8)**	**103(35.6)**	**289(100)**

Table 11.10 shows the sector of employment and level of psychological well-being the psychological well-being of MDR-TB patients according to their type of employment sector. The patients who were employed in the Government sector were 5.9 per cent,

among them there is no low level of psychological well-being, 5,5 per cent of them had evidence of a Moderate level of psychological well-being and 0.3 per cent of them had a high level of psychological well-being. The patients who were employed in the private sector were 8 per cent, among them 2.8 per cent of them had a low level of psychological well-being, 5.2 per cent of them had evidence of a Moderate level of psychological well-being and there is no high level of psychological well-being.

The patients who were working as Labour/daily wages were 25.3 per cent, among them 1.7 per cent of them had a low level of psychological well-being 11.4 per cent of them had evidence of Moderate level of psychological well-being and 12.1 per cent of them had a high level of psychological well-being. The patients who were working as self-employed were 5.2 per cent, among them 0.3 per cent of them had a low level of psychological well-being2.8 per cent of them had evidence of a Moderate level of psychological well-being and 2.1 per cent of them had a high level of psychological well-being.

The other 55.7 per cent of patients did not fit into any of the above categories, and 4.2 per cent of them had a low level of psychological well-being. 31.8 per cent of them showed evidence of moderate psychological well-being, while 19.7% showed signs of strong psychological well-being. MDR-TB patients who worked as labour/daily wage were (25.3 per cent) and among them (11.4 per cent) had evidence of a moderate level of psychological well-being, whereas MDR-TB patients who did not work at all were (55.7 per cent) and more than one-third (31.8 per cent) had evidence of the moderate level of psychological well-being.

Table 11.11: Monthly Income and Level of Psychological Well-being

Sl. No.	*Monthly Income*	*Level of Psychological Well-being*			*Total*
		Low	*Moderate*	*High*	
1.	2000 to 5000	4(21.1)(1.4)	27(16.2)(9.3)	23(22.3)(8.0)	54(18.7)
2.	5001 to 10000	2(10.5)(0.7)	21(12.6)(7.3)	21(20.4)(7.3)	44(15.2)
3.	above 10000	1(5.3)(0.3)	26(15.6)(9.0)	2(1.9)(0.7)	29(10.0)
4.	Not Applicable	12(63.2)(4.2)	93(55.7)(32.2)	57(55.3)(19.7)	162(56.1)
	Total	**19(6.6)**	**167(57.8)**	**103(35.6)**	**289(100)**

The association between monthly income and the level of psychological well-being of MDR-TB patients is shown in Table 11.11 Patients with a monthly income of up to Rs. 5000/- per month accounted for 18.7% of the total, with (1.4%) having a low level of psychological well-being, (9.3%) having a moderate level of psychological well-being, and 8% having a high level of psychological well-being.

Patients with a monthly income of Rs. 5001 to 10000 were 15.2 per cent more likely to have a low level of psychological well-being. 0.7 per cent had evidence of moderate or high psychological well-being, while 7.3 per cent in the same income category had evidence of moderate or high psychological well-being.

Patients with a monthly income of more than Rs. 10,000 were 10%, and those with a low level of psychological well-being were 0.3 per cent. Those with a moderate level of psychological well-being were 9%, and those with a high level of psychological well-being were 0.7 per cent.

As seen in the table above, more than half of the respondents (56.1%) were not eligible for any type of income. In this group, 4, 2 per cent of the patients had a low level of psychological well-being, 32.2 per cent had a moderate level of psychological well-being, and 19.7% had a high level of psychological well-being.

According to the data, more than half of MDR-TB patients (56.1%) had no income, whereas 32.2 per cent had a moderate level of psychological well-being, which showed indications of a moderately positive relationship with their income level. MDR-TB patients were unable to work regularly due to the extended duration and unanticipated outcomes.

Table 11.12: Feeling about Disease and Level of Psychological Well-being

Sl. No.	*Feeling About Disease*	*Level of Psychological Well-being*			*Total*
		Low	*Moderate*	*High*	
1.	Better	8(42.1)(2.8)	68(40.7)(23.5)	44(42.7)(15.2)	120(41.5)
2.	Same	6(31.6)(2.1)	66(39.5)(22.8)	37(35.9)(12.8)	109(37.7)
3.	Worsen	2(10.5)(0.7)	16(9.6)(5.5)	13(12.6)(4.5)	31(10.7)
4.	No Response	3(15.8)(1.0)	17(10.2)(5.9)	9(8.7)(3.1)	29(10.0)
Total		**19(6.6)**	**167(57.8)**	**103(35.6)**	**289(100)**

Table 11.12 depicts the relationship between MDR-TB patients' perceptions of their disease and their psychological well-being. Patients who had a better attitude toward their disease made up 41.5 per cent of the group, while those who had a low level of psychological well-being made up 2.8 per cent. 23,5 per cent of this group had evidence of a moderate level of psychological well-being, while 15.2% had evidence of a low level of psychological well-being.

Patients with the same feelings about the condition were (37.7%). 2.1 per cent had a low level of psychological well-being, 22.8 per cent had evidence of a moderate level of psychological well-being, and 12.8 per cent had a high level of psychological well-being. Patients with worsening feelings about their illness made up 10.7%, while those with a low degree of psychological well-being made up 0.7%, those with a moderate level of 5.5 per cent, and those with a high level of 4.5 per cent. 10% of patients had no response to their sentiments about the disease. One per cent had a poor sense of purpose, 5.9% had a moderate sense of purpose, and 3.1% had a high sense of purpose. In the table above, individuals who felt better with the disease were fewer than half (41.5%), with around one-quarter feeling better and (23.5%) having evidence of a moderate degree of psychological well-being based on their better feelings about the disease.

Table 11.13: Kind of Problem and Level of Psychological Well-being

Sl. No.	*What Kind of Problem*	*Level of Psychological Well-being*			*Total*
		Low	*Moderate*	*High*	
1.	Toxic Side effects	5(26.3)(1.7)	22(13.2)(7.6)	15(14.6)(5.2)	42(14.5)
2.	Economical	5(26.3)(1.7)	46(27.5)(15.9)	30(29.1)(10.4)	81(28.0)
3.	Social	1(5.3)(0.3)	15(9.0)(5.2)	11(10.7)(3.8)	27(9.3)
4.	Others	8(42.1)(2.8)	84(50.3)(29.1)	47(45.6)(16.3)	139(48.1)
	Total	**19(6.6)**	**167(57.8)**	**103(35.6)**	**289(100)**

The association between the type of problem and MDR-TB patients' psychological well-being is shown in Table 11.13. Toxic side effects affected 14.5 per cent of the patients, while low psychological well-being affected 4.2 per cent. Of this group, 14.5 per cent exhibited evidence of moderate psychological well-being, while (2.1 per cent) showed evidence of high psychological well-being.

Patients with financial difficulties accounted for 28% of the total, whereas those with low psychological well-being (5.9%), moderate level of psychological well-being (18%), and high psychological well-being (4.2%) were found. Patients with social problems accounted for 9.3% of the total, whereas those with low psychological well-being (0.3%), moderate level of psychological well-being (5.2%), and high psychological well-being (3.8%) were found.

The type of problem and level of psychological well-being can be determined from the table above. Patients with drug-resistant tuberculosis (MDR-TB). Twenty-eight per cent of individuals surveyed had financial difficulties, while 15.9% of those surveyed had a moderate level of psychological distress. Patients with additional issues accounted for 48.1 per cent of the total, with 29.1 per cent displaying signs of moderate psychological distress.

Table 11.14: Family Support and Level of Psychological Well-being

Sl. No.	*Family Member Support*	*Level of Psychological Well-being*			*Total*
		Low	*Moderate*	*High*	
1.	Yes	3(15.8)(1.0)	45(26.9)(15.6)	23(22.3)(8.0)	71(24.6)
2.	No	16(84.2)(5.5)	122(73.1)(42.2)	80(77.7)(27.7)	218(75.4)
Total		**19(6.6)**	**167(57.8)**	**103(35.6)**	**289(100)**

The association between family member support and self-acceptance among MDR-TB patients is shown in Table 11.14. There was 24.6 per cent of patients who had family member support, 1% of patients who had evidence of a low degree of self-acceptance, 15.6 per cent of patients who had evidence of a moderate level of psychological wellness, and 8% of patients who had evidence of a high level of psychological well-being in the patient group.

Family members supported the patient group in 75.4 per cent of cases, (5.5 per cent) had a low degree of self-acceptance, (42.2 per cent) had a moderate level of psychological wellness, and (27.7%) had a high level of psychological well-being. The support and psychological well-being of MDR-TB patients' family members have been discovered.

One-quarter of the patients (24.6%) received support from family members, and 15.6 per cent demonstrated signs of moderate psychological well-being. Seventy-four per cent (75.4%) of the patients said they had received no help from family members, whereas 42.2% had a moderate level of psychological well-being.

Table 11.15: Level of Self-Acceptance

Sl. No.	*Level of Self-Acceptance*	*Frequency*	*per cent*
1.	Low	45	15.6
2.	Moderate	170	58.8
3.	High	74	25.6
Total		**289**	**100**

The Level of Self-Acceptanceis shown in Table 11.15, Low levels of self-acceptance were observed in 15.6 per cent of MDR-TB patients. A moderate level of self-acceptance strikes 58.8% of patients, whereas a high level of self-acceptance affects 25.6 per cent. The majority of MDR-TB patients have a Moderate level Level of Self-Acceptance according to data.

Table 11.16: Sex and Level of Self-Acceptance

Sl. No.	*Sex*	*Level of Self-Acceptance*			*Total*
		Low	*Moderate*	*High*	
1.	Male	35(77.8)(12.1)	116(68.2)(40.1)	59(79.7)(20.4)	210(72.7)
2.	Female	10(22.2)(3.5)	54(31.8)(18.7)	15(20.3)(5.2)	79(27.3)
Total		**45(15.6)**	**170(58.8)**	**74(25.6)**	**289(100)**

Table 11.16 shows the sex and level of psychological well-being of MDR-TB patients. The respondents were those who were male. 72.7 per cent, among them (12.1%) had a low level of self-acceptance. However, evidence of a moderate level of psychological well-being was noticed among (40.1%) per cent of the patients and 20.4% per cent of the patients had a high level of self-acceptance. The respondents who were female were 27.3 per cent. Among them, (3.5%) had a low level of self-acceptance. However, evidence of a moderate level of psychological well-being was noticed among

(18.7%) of the patients and (5.2%) cent of the patients had a high level of self-acceptance.

The majority of the respondents (72.7%) were male, and there was evidence of a moderate level of self-acceptance with almost half (40.1%) of the respondents reporting a level of self-acceptance. When compared to females, 27.3 per cent among them, there is evidence of a moderate level of psychological well-being was noticed (18.7).

Table 11.17: Age and Level of Self-Acceptance

S. No.	*Age of the Patients*	*Level of Self-Acceptance*			*Total*
		Low	*Moderate*	*High*	
1.	18 to 30 years	9(20.0)(3.1)	42(24.7)(14.5)	20(27.0)(6.9)	71(24.6)
2.	31 to 40 years	8(17.8)(2.8)	26(15.3)(9.0)	8(10.8)(2.8)	42(14.5)
3.	41 to 50 years	10(22.2)(3.5)	40(23.5)(13.8)	15(20.3)(5.2)	65(22.5)
4.	51 to 60 years	10(22.2)(3.5)	38(22.4)(13.1)	25(33.8)(8.7)	73(25.3)
5.	Above 60 years	8(17.8)(2.8)	24(14.1)(8.3)	6(8.1)(2.1)	38(13.1)
Total		**45(15.6)**	**170(58.8)**	**74(25.6)**	**289(100)**

Table 11.17 shows the age and level of self-acceptance of MDR-TB patients according to their age. The patients who were age between 18 to 30 years were 24.6 per cent, among them (3.1%) of them had a low level of self-acceptance. (14.5) per cent of them had a Moderate Level of Self-Acceptance and (6.9%) per cent of them had a high level of self-acceptance.

The patients who were aged between 31 and 40 years were 14.5 per cent. Among them, (2.8%) of them had a low level of self-acceptance, (9.0) of cent had evidence of a moderate level of self-acceptance and (2.8%) of them had a high level of self-acceptance. The patients who were aged between 41 to 50 years were 22.5 per cent. Among them, (3.5%) cent of them had a low level of self-acceptance, 13.8 per cent of them had a moderate level of self-acceptance and (5.2%) of them had a high level of self-acceptance.

The patients who were aged between 51 to 60 years were 25.3 per cent. Among them, 3.5 per cent of them had a low level of self-acceptance, (13.1%) per cent of them had a moderate level of self-acceptance and (8.7%) of them had a high level of self-acceptance.

The patients who were aged above 60 years were 13.1 per cent. Among them, 2.8 per cent of them had a low level of self-acceptance, 8.3 per cent of them had a moderate level of self-acceptance and (2.1%) of them had a high level of self-acceptance. It is observed that the patients who were age between 18 to 30 years were (24.6) and among them, (14.5) per cent of them had a Moderate level of self-acceptance and the patients who were age between 51 to 60 years were (25.3%) and among them (13.8) per cent of them had Moderate Level of Self-Acceptance.

Table 11.18: Religion and Level of Self-Acceptance

Sl. No	*Religion*	*Level of Self-Acceptance*			*Total*
		Low	*Moderate*	*High*	
1.	Hindu	42(93.3)(14.5)	155(91.2)(53.6)	68(91.9)(23.5)	265(91.7)
2.	Muslim	2(4.4)(0.7)	11(6.5)(3.8)	3(4.1)(1.0)	16(5.5)
3.	Christian	1(2.2)(0.3)	4(2.4)(1.4)	3(4.1)(1.0)	8(2.8)
Total		**45(15.6)**	**170(58.8)**	74(25.6)	**289(100)**

Table 11.18 shows the Religion and level of Self-Acceptance of MDR-TB patients according to their religion. The patients who belong to Hindu were (91.7%) per cent, among them (14.5%) of them had a low level of Self-Acceptance, however evidence of Moderate level of Self-Acceptance was noticed among 53.6 per cent, (23.5%) per cent of them had a high level of Self-Acceptance.

The patients who belong to the Muslim religion were (5.5) per cent, among them 0.7 per cent of them had a low level of Self-Acceptance 3.8 per cent of them had evidence of Moderate level of Self-Acceptance and one per cent of them had a high level of Self-Acceptance.

The patients who belong to Christian were 2.8 per cent, among them 0.3 per cent of them had a low level of Self-Acceptance, 1.4 per cent of them had a Moderate level of Self-Acceptance and one per cent had a high level of Self.

Table 11.19 shows that the level of Self-Acceptance in the psychological well-being of MDR-TB patients according to their educational qualification. 7.3 per cent of the MDR-TB patients were

Illiterate, among them 0.3 per cent of them had a low level of Self-Acceptance (5.5%) of them had evidence of Moderatelevel of Self-Acceptance and 1.4 per cent of them had a high level of Self-Acceptance.

Table 11.19: Education and Level of Self-Acceptance

Sl. No.	*Education*	*Level of Self-Acceptance*			*Total*
		Low	*Moderate*	*High*	
1.	Illiterate	1(2.2)(0.3)	16(9.4)(5.5)	4(5.4)(1.4)	21(7.3)
2.	Primary level	9(20.0)(3.1)	35(20.6)(12.1)	16(21.6)(5.5)	60(20.8)
3.	High School	14(31.1)(4.8)	58(34.1)(20.1)	24(32.4)(8.3)	96(33.2)
4.	Higher Secondary	9(20.0)(3.1)	29(17.1)(10.0)	19(25.7)(6.6)	57(19.7)
5.	Under graduation	6(13.3)(2.1)	18(10.6)(6.2)	5(6.8)(1.7)	29(10.0)
6.	Post graduation	4(8.9)(1.4)	10(5.9)(3.5)	4(5.4)(1.4)	18(6.2)
7.	Others	2(4.4)(0.7)	4(2.4)(1.4)	2(2.7)(0.7)	8(2.8)
Total		**45(15.6)**	**170(58.8)**	**74(25.6)**	**289(100)**

The patients who were primary educational qualification were 20.8 per cent, among them 3.1 per cent of them had a low level of Self-Acceptance, (12.1%) per cent of them had evidence of Moderatelevel of Self-Acceptance and 5.5 per cent of them had a high level of Self-Acceptance. The patients who completed High school were 33.2 per cent, among them 4.8 per cent of them had a low level of Self-Acceptance, 20.1 per cent of them had evidence of Moderatelevel of Self-Acceptance and 8.3 per cent of them had a high level of Self-Acceptance. 19.7 per cent of the MDR-TB patients were completed higher secondary, among them 3.1 per cent of them had a low level of Self-Acceptance, ten per cent of them had evidence of Moderate level of Self-Acceptance and 6.6 per cent of them and had the level of Self-Acceptance. The patients who studied up to under graduation were ten per cent, among them 2.1 per cent of them had a low level of Self-Acceptance and (6.2%) of them had evidence of Moderate level of Self-Acceptance and 1.4 per cent of them had a high level of Self-Acceptance.

The patients who studied up to postgraduation were 6.2 per cent, among them 1.4 per cent of them had a low level of Self-Acceptance,

3.5 per cent of them had evidence of a Moderate level of Self-Acceptance and 1.4 per cent of the high level of Self-Acceptance. The patients those who studied other qualification were 2.8 per cent, among them 0.7 per cent of them had a low level of Self-Acceptance, 1.4 per cent evidence of Moderate level of Self-Acceptance and there is 0.7 per cent of them had a high level of Self-Acceptance. It is observed that those who have studied up to High school were 33.2 per cent Among them nearly one fifth (20.1%) of them having evidence of the level of Self-Acceptance where as who have studied up to under graduation were ten per cent among them 6.2 per cent of them having evidence of the level of Self-Acceptance.

Table 11.20: Marital Status and Level of Self-Acceptance

Sl. No.	*Marital Status*	*Level of Self-Acceptance*			*Total*
		Low	*Moderate*	*High*	
1.	Unmarried	8(17.8)(2.8)	36(21.2)(12.5)	16(21.6)(5.5)	60(20.8)
2.	Married	32(71.1)(11.1)	116(68.2)(40.1)	52(70.3)(18.0)	200(69.2)
3.	Separated	3(6.7)(1.0)	5(2.9)(1.7)	3(4.1)(1.0)	11(3.8)
4.	Widow/er	2(4.4)(0.7)	13(7.6)(4.5)	3(4.1)(1.0)	18(6.2)
	Total	**45(15.6)**	**170(58.8)**	**74(25.6)**	**289(100)**

Table 11.20 shows that the level of self-acceptance psychological well-being of MDR-TB patients according to their Marital Status. Unmarried MDR-TB patients were 20.8 per cent, among them 2.8 per cent of them had a low level of self-acceptance, 12.5 per cent of them had evidence of a moderate level of self-acceptance and 5.5 per cent of them and had a high level of self-acceptance. Of the patients who were married 69.2 per cent, among them 11.1 per cent of them had a low level of self-acceptance, (40.1%) of them had evidence of a moderate level of self-acceptance and 18p er cent of them had a high level of self-acceptance. The patients who were separated were 3.8, among them one per cent of them had a low level of self-acceptance, 1.7 per cent of them had evidence of a moderate level of self-acceptance and one per cent of them had a high level of self-acceptance.

The patients who were Widow/er 6.2 per cent, among them 0.7 per cent of them had a low level of self-acceptance, 4.5 per cent of them had evidence of a moderate level of self-acceptance and one per cent of the high level of self-acceptance among the widow/er participants. It is observed that the patients who were married were 69.2 per cent and among this group majority, (40.1%) of them had the evidence of Moderate level of self-acceptance whereas the unmarried patients were (20.8%), among them (12.5) per cent of them had Moderate level of self-acceptance.

Table 11.21: Type of Family and Level of Self-Acceptance

Sl. No.	*Type of Family*	*Level of Self-Acceptance*			*Total*
		Low	*Moderate*	*High*	
1.	Joint Family	7(15.6)(2.4)	15(8.8)(5.2)	11(14.9)(3.8)	33(11.4)
2.	Nuclear Family	35(77.8)(12.1)	147(86.5)(50.9)	58(78.4)(20.1)	240(83.0)
3.	Not Applicable	3(6.7)(1.0)	8(4.7)(2.8)	5(6.8)(1.7)	16(5.5)
Total		**45(15.6)**	**170(58.8)**	**74(25.6)**	**28(100)**

Table 11.21 shows the Type of family and level of self-acceptance according to their type of family. The patients who were living in the joint families were 11.4 per cent, among them 2.4 per cent of them had a low level of self-acceptance, 5.2 per cent of them had evidence of a moderate level of self-acceptance and 3.8 per cent of them had a high level of self-acceptance. The patients who were living in the nuclear family were 83 per cent, among them 12.1 per cent of them had a low level of self-acceptance, 50.9 per cent of them had evidence of a moderate level of self-acceptance and 20.1 per cent of them had a high level of self-acceptance.

The remaining 5.5 per cent of them living with friends and hostel etc which was not applicable, among them one per cent of them had a low level of self-acceptance, 2.8 per cent of them had a moderate level of self-acceptance and 1.7 per cent of them had a high level of self-acceptance.

It is observed from the above table the type of family and level of self-acceptance of the MDR-TB patient's the majority 83% of them living in the nuclear family, among them half (50.9%) of them had evidence of a moderate level of self-acceptance, when compared to the joint family were 11.4 per cent, among them the evidence of Moderate level of self-acceptance had only 5.2 per cent, this shows that the joint family had the family support in connection with the level of self-acceptance.

Table 11.22: Number of Family Members and Level of Self-Acceptance

S. No.	*Number of Family Members*	*Level of Self-Acceptance*			*Total*
		Low	*Moderate*	*High*	
1.	One	2(4.4)(0.7)	10(5.9)(3.5)	6(8.1)(2.1)	18(6.2)
2.	Two	19(42.2)(6.6)	70(41.2)(24.2)	22(29.7)(7.6)	111(38.4)
4.	Above 5	3(6.7)(1.0)	4(2.4)(1.4)	6(8.1)(2.1)	13(4.5)
Total		45(15.6)	170(58.8)	74(25.6)	289(100)

Table 11.22 shows the number of family members living with them and the level of self-acceptance of the MDR-TB patients. The patients who were living with one family member were 6.2 per cent, among them 0.7 per cent of them had a level of self-acceptance 3.5 per cent of them had evidence of a moderate level of self-acceptance and 2.1 per cent of them had a high level of self-acceptance. The patients who were living with two members in the family were 38.4 per cent, among them (6.6) per cent of them had a level of self-acceptance, 24.2 per cent of them had evidence of a moderate level of self-acceptance and 7.6 per cent of them had a high level of self-acceptance.

The patients who were living with 3 to 5 members in the family were 50.9 per cent, among them 12.1 per cent of them had a low level of self-acceptance, 30.4 per cent of them had evidence of a moderate level of self-acceptance and (8.3) per cent of them had a level of self-acceptance. The patients who were living with above 5 members in the family were 4.5 per cent, among them one per cent of them had a low level of self-acceptance1.4 per cent of them had evidence of a moderate level of self-acceptance and there is evidence of a high level of self-acceptance were 2.1 per cent among above 5 members living in the family.

It is observed that from the above table half of the MDR-TB patients (50.9%) were living with 3 to 5 family members, among them there is evidence of a moderate level of self-acceptance of 31.5 per cent in the psychological well-being of MDR-TB patients.

Table 11.23: Employment Status and Level of Self-Acceptance

S. No.	*Employment Status*	*Level of Self-Acceptance*			*Total*
		Low	*Moderate*	*High*	
1.	Employed	23(51.1)(8.0)	73(42.9)(25.3)	32(43.2)(11.1)	128(44.3)
2.	Unemployed	15(33.3)(5.2)	66(38.8)(22.8)	29(39.2)(10.0)	110(38.1)
3.	Student	3(6.7)(1.0)	21(12.4)(7.3)	6(8.1)(2.1)	30(10.4)
4.	Housewife	4(8.9)(1.4)	10(5.9)(3.5)	7(9.5)(2.4)	21(7.3)
	Total	**45(15.6)**	**170(58.8)**	**74(25.6)**	**289(100)**

Table 11.23 shows the level of self-acceptance of MDR-TB patients according to their workplace. The patients who were employed were 44.3 per cent, among them eight per cent of them had a low level of self-acceptance 25.3 per cent of them had evidence of a moderate level of self-acceptance and 11.1 per cent of them had a high low level of self-acceptance. The unemployed patients were 38.1 per cent, among them 5.2 per cent of them had a low low level of self-acceptance, 22.8 per cent of them had evidence of a moderate level of self-acceptance and ten per cent of them had a high low level of self-acceptance. The patients those who were student were 10.4 per cent, among them one per cent of them had a low low level of self-acceptance, 7.3 per cent of them had evidence of a moderate level of self-acceptance and (2.1%) of them had a high low level of self-acceptance.

The patients those who were housewife were 7.3 per cent, among them 1.4 per cent of them had a low low level of self-acceptance, (3.5%) of them had evidence of a moderate level of self-acceptance and there is 2.4 per cent of them had a high low level of self-acceptance according to the above table, MDR-TB patients who were employed (44.3%) among them(25.3%) had evidence of a moderate level of self-acceptance, whereas MDR-TB patients who were unemployed (38.1%) among the unemployed (22.8%) had evidence of a moderate level of self-acceptance.

Table 11.24 shows the type of employment and level of self-acceptance of MDR-TB patients according to their type of employment sector. The patients who were employed in the Government sector were 5.9 per cent, among them one per cent of them had a low level of self-acceptance, 3.8 per cent of them had evidence of a moderate level of self-acceptance and one per cent of them had a high level of self-acceptance.

Table 11.24: Type of Employment and Level of Self-Acceptance

Sl. No.	*Type of Employment*	*Level of Self-Acceptance*			*Total*
		Low	*Moderate*	*High*	
1.	Government	3(6.7)(1.0)	11(6.5)(3.8)	3(4.1)(1.0)	17(5.9)
2.	Private	4(8.9)(1.4)	13(7.6)(4.5)	6(8.1)(2.1)	23(8.0)
3.	Labour/daily wages	12(26.7)(4.2)	39(22.9)(13.5)	22(29.7)(7.6)	73(25.3)
4.	Self Employed	4(8.9)(1.4)	10(5.9)(3.5)	1(1.4)(0.3)	15(5.2)
5.	Not Applicable	22(48.9)(7.6)	97(57.1)(33.6)	42(56.8)(14.5)	161(55.7)
Total		**45(15.6)**	**170(58.8)**	**74(25.6)**	**289(100)**

The patients who were employed in the private sector were 8 per cent, among them 1.4 per cent of them had a low level of self-acceptance, 4.5 per cent of them had evidence of a moderate level of self-acceptance and 2.1 per cent of them had a high level of self-acceptance.

The patients who were working as labour/daily wages were 25.3 per cent. Among them, 4.2 per cent had a low level of self-acceptance. 13.5 per cent of them had evidence of a moderate level of self-acceptance and 7.6 per cent of them had a high level of self-acceptance.

The patients who were working as self-employed were 5.2 per cent, among them 1.4 per cent of them had a low level of self-acceptance 3.5 per cent of them had evidence of a Moderate level of self-acceptance and 0.3 per cent of them had a high level of self-acceptance.

The remaining patients who were not applying any of the above categories were 55.7 per cent, among them 7.6 per cent of them had a low level of self-acceptance33.6 per cent of them had evidence of a

Moderate level of self-acceptance and 14.5 per cent of them had a high level of self-acceptance.

In the above table, MDR-TB patients who worked as labour/daily wage were (25.3%) and among them (13.5%) had evidence of a moderate level of the purpose of life, whereas MDR-TB patients who did not work any were (55.7%) and among them, more than one-third (33.6%) had evidence of a moderate level of the purpose of life.

Table 11.25: Monthly Income and Level of Self-Acceptance

S. No.	*Monthly Income*	*Level of Self-Acceptance*			*Total*
		Low	*Moderate*	*High*	
1.	Up to 5000	12(26.7)(4.2)	32(18.8)(11.1)	10(13.5)(3.5)	54(18.7)
2.	5001 to 10000	6(13.3)(2.1)	23(13.5)(8.0)	15(20.3)(5.2)	44(15.2)
3.	above 10000	5(11.1)(1.7)	17(10.0)(5.9)	7(9.5)(2.4)	29(10.0)
4.	Not Applicable	22(48.9)(7.6)	98(57.6)(33.9)	42(56.8)(14.5)	162(56.1)
	Total	45(15.6)	170(58.8)	74(25.6)	**289(100.0)**

Table 11.25 shows the relationship between the Monthly income and level of self-acceptance of MDR-TB patients. The patient group those who were earning monthly income up to Rs. 5000/- per month were 18.7 per cent, among them those who were the low level of self-acceptance were (4.2%), among this income group (11.1%) of them had evidence of a moderate level of self-acceptance and 3.5 per cent of the patients had a high level of self-acceptance.

The patients who were in the monthly income between Rs. 5001 to 10000 were 15.2 per cent among them who had a low level of self-acceptance were 2.1 per cent, in the same income group eight per cent had evidence of a moderate level of self-acceptance and 5.2 per cent had a high level of self-acceptance.

The patients who were in the monthly income above 10000 were ten per cent, among them who had a low level of self-acceptance were 1.7 per cent, in the same income group 5.9 per cent had evidence of a moderate level of self-acceptance and 2. 4 per cent had a high level of self-acceptance.

It is evident from the above table more than half (56.1%) of the respondents were not eligible for any income. In this category 7.6 per cent of them were a low level of self-acceptance, 33.9 per cent had evidence of a moderate level of self-acceptance and 14.5 per cent of the patients had a high level of self-acceptance.

According to the preceding statistics, more than half of the MDR-TB patients (56.1%) had no income, whereas 33.9 per cent revealed evidence of the somewhat positive connection with their income level. Due to the longer duration and unexpected consequences, MDR-TB patients were unable to work regularly.

Table 11.26: Feeling About Disease and Level of Self-Acceptance

Sl. No.	*Feeling about Disease*	*Level of Self-Acceptance*			*Total*
		Low	*Moderate*	*High*	
1.	Better	18(40.0)(6.2)	71(41.8)(24.6)	31(41.9)(10.7)	120(41.5)
2.	Same	11(24.4)(3.8)	65(38.2)(22.5)	33(44.6)(11.4)	109(37.7)
3.	Worsen	10(22.2)(3.5)	15(8.8)(5.2)	6(8.1)(2.1)	31(10.7)
4.	No Response	6(13.3)(2.1)	19(11.2)(6.6)	4(5.4)(1.4)	29(10.0)
Total		45(15.6)	170(58.8)	74(25.6)	**289(100)**

The link between MDR-TB patients' feelings about their condition and their level of self-acceptance is shown in Table 11.26. Patients with a better feeling toward their disease made up 41.5 per cent of the group, and those with a low level of self-acceptance made up 6.2 per cent, 24.6 per cent of this group had evidence of a moderate level of self-acceptance, and (10.7%) had evidence of a low level of self-acceptance.

The patients who had the same feelings about the illness were (36.7%). Among them, 3.8 per cent had a low level of self-acceptance, 22.5 per cent had evidence of a moderate level of self-acceptance, and (11.4%) per cent had a high level of self-acceptance.

Patients with worsening feelings about their illness comprised (10.7%), those with a low level of self-acceptance comprised 3.5 per cent, those with a moderate level of self-acceptance made up 5.2 per cent, and those with a high level of self-acceptance made up 2.1 per cent.10 per cent of the patients had no response to their feelings about the disease, 2.1 per cent had a level of self-acceptance of life, 6.6% had a moderate level of self-acceptance, and (1.4%) had a high level of self-acceptance.

It is noteworthy that in the table above the relationship between disease sensitivity and the positive relationship of MDR-TB patients, those who felt better with the disease were less than half (41.5%), of whom about one-fourth felt better and (24.6%) had evidence of a Moderate level of self-acceptance according to of their better feelings about the disease.

It is observed that Patients who had similar feelings about the disease were (37.7%) among them, about one-fourth of them (22.5%) per cent had evidence of a moderate level of self-acceptance, according to their similar feelings about the disease

Table 11.27: Kind of Problem and Level of Self-Acceptance

Sl. No.	*What kind of Problem*	*Level of Self-Acceptance*			*Total*
		Low	*Moderate*	*High*	
1.	Toxic Side effects	10(22.2)(3.5)	21(12.4)(7.3)	11(14.9)(3.8)	42(14.5)
2.	Economical	13(28.9)(4.5)	46(27.1)(15.9)	22(29.7)(7.6)	81(28.0)
3.	Social	5(11.1)(1.7)	17(10.0)(5.9)	5(6.8)(1.7)	27(9.3)
4.	Others	17(37.8)(5.9)	86(50.6)(29.8)	36(48.6)(12.5)	139(48.1)
Total		**45(15.6)**	**170(58.8)**	**74(25.6)**	**289(100)**

The kind of difficult MDR-TB therapy and the level of self-acceptance among MDR-TB patients are shown in Table 11.27. According to the above table, 14.5% of the patients had toxic side effects from MDR-TB treatment, and 3.5% of them showed a low level of self-acceptance, 7.3% showed a moderate level of self-acceptance, and the remaining 3.8% showed a high level of self-acceptance.

Patients experiencing financial difficulties while taking MDR-TB treatment made up 28% of the total, with 4.5 per cent having a low level of self-acceptance, 5.9 per cent having a moderate level of self-acceptance, and 1.7 per cent having a high level of self-acceptance. Patients having social problems during MDR-TB treatment were 9.3 per cent of the total, with 1.7 per cent having a low level of self-acceptance, 5.9 per cent having a moderate level of self-acceptance, and 1.7 showing a high level of self-acceptance.

In addition to side-effects, economic and social issues during the treatment of MDR-TB, 5.9 per cent of the patients had a low level of self-acceptance, 29.8 per cent had a moderate level of self-acceptance and the remainder, 12.5 had a high level of self-acceptance, the table above shows.

Table 11.28: Family Support and Level of Self-Acceptance

S. No.	*Family Member Support*	*Level of Self-Acceptance*			*Total*
		Low	*Moderate*	*High*	
1.	Yes	5(11.1)(1.7)	46(27.1)(15.9)	20(27.0)(6.9)	71(24.6)
2.	No	40(88.9)(13.8)	124(72.9)(42.9)	54(73.0)(18.7)	218(75.4)
	Total	**45(15.6)**	**170(58.8)**	**74(25.6)**	**289(100)**

Table 11.28 shows the relationship between family member support and the level of self-acceptance among MDR-TB patients. The patient group included 24.6 per cent who had family member support, 1.7 per cent who had evidence of a low level of self-acceptance, 15.9 per cent who had evidence of a moderate level of self-acceptance, and 6.9% had evidence of a high level of self-acceptance.

The patient group had (75.4%) support from family members, (13.8%) had a low level of self-acceptance, (42.9%) had a moderate level of self-acceptance, and (18.7%) had a high level of self-acceptance. It has been found that the support and level of self-acceptance of MDR-TB patients' family members. One-fourth of the patients (24.6%) had family member support, and 15.9 per cent showed evidence of a somewhat positive relationship. Three-quarters (75.4%) of the patients reported no assistance from family members, whereas 42.9 per cent had a moderate level of self-acceptance.

CHAPTER 12

General Health Status of MDR-TB Patients

This part provides an overall health state of MDR-TB patients using the general health questionnaire (GHQ12), which comprises 12 items and is analysed using a Likert scale to diagnose mental problems. The variables listed below are being examined. Consideration should be given to characteristics such as state, gender, age, religion, educational qualifications, family type, patient employment, and marital status. This part assesses the (your) general health to see if they (you) are experiencing physical or psychological suffering.

Table 12.1: Age and Level of the General Health of MDR-TB Patients

Sl. No.	*Age of the Patients*	*Level of General Health*			*Total*
		Normal	*Evidence of Distress*	*Severe Problems*	
1.	18 to 30 years	11(19.0)(3.8)	19(25.7)(6.6)	41(26.1)(14.2)	71(24.6)
2.	31 to 40 years	13(22.4)(4.5)	11(14.9)(3.8)	18(11.5)(6.2)	42(14.5)
3.	41 to 50 years	15(25.9(5.2)	14(18.9)(4.8)	36(22.9)(12.5)	65(22.5)
4.	51 to 60 years	16(27.6)(5.5)	11(14.9)(3.8)	46(29.3)(5.9)	73(25.3)
5.	Above 60 years	3(5.2)(1.0)	19(25.7)(6.6)	16(10.2)(5.5)	38(13.1)
Total		**58(20.1)**	74(25.6)	**157(54.3)**	**289(100)**

The above Table 12.1 shows the age-wise distribution of MDR-TB patients with evidence of psychological distress. The respondents in the age group of 18 to 30 years of age were 24.6 per cent, among them 14.2 per cent had severe problems and psychological distress, 6.6 per cent had evidence of distress and the remaining about one third (3.8 1) did not have any distress.

The majority of the respondents who suffered psychological distress were in the age group of 18 to 30 years .70 per cent of the patients belonged to the 20–39 years age group showed that younger age groups (<40 years) were more likely to develop MDR-TB/TB and side effects than older.

The respondents in the age group of 31 to 40 years were 14.5 per cent among them 6.2 per cent of the respondents had a high level of distress and 3.8 per cent of them had evidence of distress; there was no distress among 4.5 per cent of the respondents.

The respondents in the age group of 41 to 50 years constituted 22.5 per cent among them 12.5 per cent of the respondents had severe problems and psychological distress, 4.8 per cent of them had evidence of distress and 5.2 per cent of the respondents were normal.

The respondents in the age group of 51 to 60 years were 25.3 per cent among them 5.9 per cent of the respondents had a severe problem and psychological distress, 3.8 per cent of the respondents showed evidence of distress and the remaining 5.5 per cent of the respondents were normal.

The respondents were those above 60 years was negligible (13.1) among them 5.5 per cent of them had severe problems and psychological distress 6.6 per cent of them had evidence of distress and the remaining one per cent of the patients were normal.

It can be observed that there is a high level (14.2) of psychological distress and evidence of distress (6.6) among the age group between 18 to 30 years, which means that young MDR-TB patients were the most affected age group.

Table 12.2: Religion and Level of General Health

Sl. No.	*The Religion of the Patients*	*Level of General Health*			*Total*
		Normal	*Evidence of Distress*	*Psychological Distress*	
1.	Hindu	55(94.8)(19.0)	70(94.6)(24.2)	140(89.2)(48.4)	265(91.7)
2.	Muslim	3(5.2)(1.0)	4(5.4)(1.4)	9(5.7)(3.1)	16(5.50)
3.	Christian	0(0.0)(0.0)	0(0.0)(0.0)	8(5.1)(2.8)	8(2.8)
	Total	**58(20.1)**	74(25.6)	**157(54.3)**	**289(100)**

Table 12.2 shows the evidence of psychological distress of MDR-TB patients according to their religion. The respondents who were

Hindus were 91.7 per cent among them (19.0) per cent of them did not have any distress, however evidence of distress was noticed among 48.4 per cent of the patients and 24.2 per cent of the patients had severe problems and psychological distress.

The respondents who were Muslims were (5.5) per cent among them (1.0) per cent were normal without any evidence of distress. It was observed that (1.4) per cent of the Muslims had evidence of distress and 3.1 per cent of them had severe problems and psychological distress.

The respondents who were Christians were 2.8 per cent, among them it was observed that 2.8 per cent had only psychological distress and there is no typical and evidence of distress among the Christians.

It can be observed that severe psychological distress and evidence of distress were high (48.4) among the respondents those who were Hindus. The majority (48.4) of the respondents who suffered psychological distress belonged to the Hindu religion.

Table 12.3: Education Qualification and Level of General Health

Sl. No.	*Educational Qualification*	*Level of General Health*			*Total*
		Normal	*Evidence of Distress*	*Psychological Distress*	
1.	Illiterate	3(5.20)(1.0)	8(10.8)(2.8)	10(6.4)(3.5)	21(7.3)
2.	Primary level	8(13.8)(2.8)	17(23.0)(5.9)	35(22.3)(12.1)	60(20.8)
3.	High School	22(37.9)(7.6)	20(27.0)(6.9)	54(34.40)(18.7)	96(33.2)
4.	Higher Secondary	16(27.6)(5.5)	15(20.3)(5.2)	26(16.6)(9.0)	57(19.7)
5.	Under graduation	3(5.2)(1.0)	8(10.8)(2.8)	18(11.5)(6.2)	29(10.0)
6.	Post graduation	3(5.2)(1.0)	4(5.4)(1.4)	11(7.0)(3.8)	18(6.2)
7.	Others	3(5.2)(1.0)	2(2.7)(0.7)	3(1.9)(1.0)	8(2.8)
Total		**58(20.1)**	**74(25.6)**	**157(54.3)**	**289(100)**

The above Table 12.3 shows the educational qualification and evidence of distress level among the MDR-TB patients. The illiterate respondents were 7.3 per cent among them 3.5 per cent of them had severe problems and psychological distress and 2.8 per cent of them had evidence of distress and the remaining one per cent of the patients did not have any distress.

The respondents who were qualified up to primary level (5th Class) were 20.8 per cent among them 12.1 per cent of them had severe problems and psychological distress, 5.9 per cent of them had evidence of distress and the remaining 2.8) per cent of them were normal.

The patients who were qualified till high school (Metric) were 33.2 per cent among them those who had severe problems and psychological distress were 18.7 per cent, 6.9 per cent of them had evidence of distress and 7.6 per cent of them were normal. The patient those who had studied up to higher secondary (12th Class) were 19.7) per cent among them 9.0) per cent of the respondents had severe problems and psychological distress, 5.2) per cent of them had evidence of distress and 5.5) per cent of them were normal without any distress.

Among the respondent's undergraduates, ten per cent among them 6.2 per cent of them had severe problems and psychological distress, 2.8) per cent of them had evidence of distress and the remaining one per cent of them were normal.

The patients who had studied up to postgraduate were 6.2) per cent among them 3.8,) per cent had severe problems and psychological distress, 1.4 per cent of them had evidence of distress and the remaining one per cent of them did not have any distress.

The patients who had other qualifications were 2.8) per cent among them one per cent had severe problems and psychological distress, 0.7) per cent of them had evidence of distress and the remaining one per cent of them did not have any distress.

Among the respondents, those who had severe problems and psychological distress were high (6.2) among the illiterates, which is supported by the book conducted by Gajanan S. Gaude *et al.*, (2014) which proved low Education status (P = 0.01) has a significant association with Tuberculosis.

Below Table 12.4 provides the details of the relationship between marital status and evidence of distress. The unmarried respondents were 20.8 per cent among them those who had severe problems and psychological distress was 12.1 per cent; evidence of distress was 5.5 per cent and 3.1 per cent of them were normal.

Table 12.4: Marital Status and Level of General Health

Sl. No.	*Marital Status*	*Level of General Health*			*Total*
		Typical	*Evidence of Distress*	*Psychological Distress*	
1.	Unmarried	9(15.5)(3.1)	16(21.6)(5.5)	35(22.3)(12.1)	60(20.8)
2.	Married	46(79.3)(15.9)	47(63.5)(16.3)	107(68.2)(37.0)	200(69.20)
3.	Separated	2(3.4)(0.7)	1(1.4)(0.3)	8(5.1)(2.8)	11(3.8)
4.	Widow/er	1(1.7)(0.3)	10(13.5)(3.5)	7(4.5)(2.4)	18(6.2)
	Total	**58(20.1)**	74(25.6)	**157(54.3)**	**289(100)**

The married respondents were 69.2 per cent among them 37.0 per cent of them had severe problems and psychological distress, 16.3) per cent of them had evidence of distress and 15.9 per cent of the patients were normal.

The majority (37.0) of them those who were married had problems and psychological distress. This is in line with the study conducted in Pakistan by Waqas *et al.*, (2012) where the high incidence of T.B in the married alarm the concerns about the spreading consequences in the population. Among the respondents, those who were separated from their spouse were 3.8 per cent among them 2.8 per cent had severe psychological distress, but there was evidence of distress among (0.3%) of the respondents and (0.7%) of them were normal.

Table 12.5: Family Type and Level of General Health

Sl No.	*Type of Family*	*Level of General Health*			*Total*
		Typical	*Evidence of Distress*	*Psychological Distress*	
1.	Joint Family	3(5.2)(1.0)	12(16.2)(4.2)	18(11.5)(6.2)	33(11.4)
2.	Nuclear Family	54(93.1)(18.7)	60(81.1)(20.8)	126(80.3)(43.6)	240(83.0)
3.	Living Separately	1(1.7)(0.3)	2(2.7)(0.7)	13(8.3)(4.5)	16(5.5)
	Total	**58(20.1)**	74(25.6)	**157(54.3)**	**289(100)**

The patients those who were widow or widower were 6.2 per cent it was observed that 2.4 per cent of them had severe problems with psychological distress, 3.5 per cent had evidence of distress and 0.3) per cent among them were normal without any evidence of distress.

Table 12.5 shows the MDR-TB patients family type about the level of psychological distress. The patients who were living in the joint family were 11.4 per cent among them 6.2 per cent of them had severe problems and psychological distress and 4.2 per cent of them had evidence of distress; the remaining one per cent of the respondents living in the joint family was normal and there was no distress.

The patients who were living in the nuclear family were 83.0 per cent among them 43.6) per cent of the respondents had severe problems and psychological distress, 20.8 per cent of them had evidence of distress and the remaining 18.7) per cent of the respondents were normal.

The patients who were living separately, neither in the joint family nor nuclear family were 5.5 per cent among them those who had severe problems and psychological distress were 4.5 per cent, there was evidence of distress among 0.7 per cent of the respondents and 0.3 per cent of them were normal without any distress.

It is observed from the above table that the MDR-TB patients those who lived in the nuclear family had more distress when compared to the patients those who lived in joint family and living separately, which showed a significant association of low socio-economic status and Tuberculosis.

Table 12.6: Employment Status and Level of General Health

Sl. No.	*Employment status*	*Level of General Health*			*Total*
		Typical	*Evidence of Distress*	*Psychological Distress*	
1.	Employed	26(44.8)(9.0)	35(47.3)(12.1)	67(42.7)(23.2)	128(44.3)
2.	Unemployed	20(34.5)(6.9)	26(35.1)(9.0)	64(40.8)(22.1)	110(38.1)
3.	Student	5(8.6)(1.7)	9(12.2)(3.1)	16(10.2)(5.5)	30(10.4)
4.	Housewife	7(12.1)(2.4)	4(5.4)(1.4)	10(6.4)(3.5)	21(7.3)
	Total	**58(20.1)**	**74(25.6)**	**157(54.3)**	**289(100)**

Table 12.6 shows the relationship between the MDR-TB patient's employment and level of distress. The respondents who were employed were 25.1 per cent among them who were normal without any distress were 9.0 per cent, among the patients employed 12.1 per cent of the patient showed evidence of distress and 23.2 per cent showed severe problems and psychological distress. One third (38.1%) of the respondents were unemployed among them 6.9 per cent of the respondents were normal without any evidence of distress, 9.0 per cent had evidence of distress and 22.1 per cent of the patients had severe problems and psychological distress.

Among the respondents 10.4 per cent were students, among them 1.7 per cent of the students were normal, 3.1 per cent had evidence of distress and 5.5 per cent of the students had severe problems with psychological distress. Among the respondent's houses wives were 7.3 per cent among them 2.4 per cent were normal without distress among these patients 1.4 per cent had evidence of distress and 3.5 per cent of them had severe problems and psychological distress. The book found that psychological distress was equally high among the employed (23.2%) and unemployed (22.1%) MDR-TB patients, which showed a significant association of low socioeconomic status and Tuberculosis.

Table 12.7: Status of Employment and Level of General Health

Sl No.	*Status of the Employment*	*Level of General Health*			*Total*
		Typical	*Evidence of Distress*	*Psychological Distress*	
1.	Government	3(5.2)(1.0)	5(6.8)(1.7)	9(5.7)(3.1)	17(5.9)
2..	Private	5(8.6)(1.7)	7(9.5)(2.4)	11(7.0)(3.8)	23(8.0)
3.	Labour/daily wages	16(27.6)(5.5)	18(24.3)(6.2)	39(24.8)(13.5)	73(25.3)
4.	Self Employed	2(3.4)(0.7)	5(6.8)(1.7)	8(5.1)(2.8)	15(5.2)
5.	Not Applicable	32(55.2)(11.1)	39(52.7)(13.5)	90(57.3)(31.1)	161(55.7)
Total		**58(20.1)**	**74(25.6)**	**157(54.3)**	**289(100)**

Table 12.7 Table shows the relationship between the Status of Employment of the MDR-TB patients and the level of distress. The

patient group those who were working in government were 5.9 per cent among them those who were normal without any distress were one per cent, among this income group 1.7 per cent of them had evidence of distress and 3.1 per cent of the patients had severe problems and psychological distress.

The patients who were working in Private were eight per cent, among them who had distress were 1.7 per cent, in the same group 2.4 per cent had evidence of distress and 3.8 per cent had severe problems and psychological distress.25.3 per cent of the MDR-TB patients were working as a Labour/daily wages were 25.3 per cent, among them those who were 5.5 per cent normal without any evidence of distress, 6.2 per cent of the patients had evidence of distress and 13.5 per cent of the respondents had severe problems and psychological distress.

In the self-employed group, the total respondents were 5.2 per cent among them 0.7 per cent of the respondents were normal without any distress among this self-employed group 1.7 per cent of the patients were having evidence of distress and the remaining 2.8 per cent had severe problems and psychological distress. It is evident from the above table more than half (55.7%) of the respondents were not eligible for any employment status. In this category, 11.1 per cent of them were without any distress, 13.5 per cent had evidence of distress and 31.1 per cent of the patients had severe problems and psychological distress.

Table 12.8: Duration of MDR-TB Treatment and Level of General Health

Sl. No.	*Duration of MDR-TB Treatment*	*Level of General Health*			*Total*
		Normal	*Evidence of Distress*	*Severe Problems and Psychological Distress*	
1.	Less than 1 year	26(44.8)(9.0)	23(31.1)(8.0)	68(43.3)(23.5)	117(40.5)
2.	1 to 2 years	32(55.2)(11.1)	51(68.9)(17.6)	89(56.7)(30.8)	172(59.5)
	Total	**58(20.1)**	**74(25.6)**	**157(54.3)**	**289(100)**

The above Table 12.8 highlights the relationship between the duration of MDR-TB treatment taken and the psychological distress among the MDR-TB patients. It is evident from the above table that the patients who have taken less than one year of treatment for MDR-TB were 40.5 per cent, among them 23.5 per cent of them had severe problems and psychological distress, 8.0) per cent of the patients had evidence of distress and the remaining 9.0 per cent of the patients were normal.

The MDR-TB patients who have taken treatment between one year to two years were 59.5) per cent, among them 30.8 per cent of had severe problems and psychological distress, 17.6 per cent of them had evidence of distress and the remaining 11.1 per cent of the patients were normal.

Table 12.9: Feeling about Disease and Level of General Health

Sl No.	*Feeling about Disease*	*Level of General Health*			*Total*
		Typical	*Evidence of Distress*	*Psychological Distress*	
1.	Better	29(50.0)(10.0)	32(43.2)(11)	59(37.6)(20.4)	120(41.5)
2.	Same	23(39.7)(8.0)	24(32.4)(8.3)	62(39.5)(21.5)	109(37.7)
3.	Worsen	3(5.2)(1.0)	5(6.8)(1.7)	23(14.6)(8.0)	31(10.7)
4.	No Response	3(5.2)(1.0)	13(17.6)(4.5)	13(8.3)(4.5)	29(10.0)
Total		**58(20.1)**	**74(25.6)**	**157(54.3)**	**289(100)**

The above Table 12.9 highlights the relationship between the feeling about disease and level of psychological distress among MDR-TB patients. It is evident from the above table that the patients who have taken treatment for MDR-TB and had a better feeling about the disease were (41.5) per cent, among them 20.4 per cent of them had severe problems and psychological distress, 11 per cent of the patients had evidence of distress and the remaining ten per cent of the patients were normal.

The patients who have taken treatment for MDR-TB and had the same feeling about the disease for MDR-TB were (37.7) per cent, among them 21.5 per cent of them had severe problems and psychological distress, 8.3 per cent of the patients had evidence of distress and the remaining eight per cent of the patients were normal.

The patients those who have taken treatment for MDR-TB they had to worsen feeling about the disease during the period of the treatment for MDR-TB were (10.7) per cent, among them eight per cent of them had severe problems and psychological distress, 1.7 per cent of the patients had evidence of distress and the remaining one per cent of the patients were normal.

The MDR-TB patients who have taken treatment for MDR-TB there is no feeling about the treatment and the disease were ten per cent, among them 4.5 per cent of them had severe problems and psychological distress and evidence of distress respectively and remaining one per cent of the patients were normal.

Table 12.10: Problem with MDR-TB Treatment and Level of General Health

Sl. No.	*Problem with MDR-TB treatment*	*Level of General Health*			*Total*
		Typical	*Evidence of Distress*	*Psychological Distress*	
1.	Yes	25(43.1)(8.7)	38(51.4)(13.1)	72(45.9)(24.9)	135(46.7)
2.	No	33(56.9)(11.4)	36(48.6)(12.5)	85(54.1)(29.4)	154(53.3)
	Total	**58(20.1)**	**74(25.6)**	**157(54.3)**	**289(100)**

Table 12.10 shows that the problem with MDR-TB treatment and level of Psychosocial distress among the MDR-TB patients. It is evident from the above table that the patients those who have problem with treatment for MDR-TB were 46.7 per cent, among them 24.9) per cent of them had severe problems and psychological distress, 13.1 per cent of the patients had evidence of distress and the remaining 8.7) per cent of the patients were normal. The patients who have no problem with treatment for MDR-TB were 53.3 per cent, among them 29.4 per cent of them had no severe problems and psychological distress, 12.5 per cent of the patients had no evidence of distress and the remaining 11.4 per cent of the patients were normal.

Table 12.11 shows that the Type of problem and level of general health among the MDR-TB patients. It is evident from the above table that the patients those who have toxic Side effects problem with treatment for MDR-TB were 14.5 per cent, among them 6.9 per cent of them had severe problems and psychological distress, 4.5 per cent of the patients had evidence of distress and the remaining 3.1 per cent of the patients were normal.

Table 12.11: Type of Problem and Level of General Health

Sl. No.	Kind of Problem	Level of General Health			Total
		Typical	Evidence of Distress	Psychological Distress	
1.	Toxic Side effects	9(15.5)(3.1)	13(17.6)(4.5)	20(12.7)(6.9)	42(14.5)
2.	Economical	18(31.0)(6.2)	24(32.4)(8.3)	39(24.8)(13.5)	81(28.0)
3.	Social	7(12.1)(2.4)	5(6.8)(1.7)	15(9.6)(5.2)	27(9.3)
4.	Others	24(41.4)(8.3)	32(43.2)(11.1)	83(52.9)(28.7)	139(48.1)
	Total	**58(20.1)**	**74(25.6)**	**157(54.3)**	**289(100)**

The patients who have a social problem during treatment for MDR-TB were twenty-eight per cent, among them 13.5 per cent of them had no severe problems and psychological distress, 8.3 per cent of the patients had no evidence of distress and the remaining 6.2 per cent of the patients were normal. The patients those who have Economical problem during treatment for MDR-TB were 9.3 per cent, among them 5.2 per cent of them had no severe problems and psychological distress1.7 per cent of the patients had no evidence of distress and the remaining 2.4 per cent of the patients were normal. It is evident from the above table that the patients who had other problems apart from side effects, economic and social problems during treatment for MDR-TB were 48.1 per cent, among them 28.7 per cent of them had severe problems and psychological distress, 11.1 per cent of the patients had evidence of distress and the remaining 8.3 per cent of the patients were normal.

CHAPTER 13

Internalized Stigma and Mental Well-being of MDR-TB Patients

This section concentrates on the MDR-TB patient's stigma profile. The authors looks at age, gender, religion, social status, education, marital status, family status, employment status, patient monthly income, type of house, TB problem, feeling of isolation, patient sleeping pattern, patient food with family members, the patient uses separate utensils and the state where the patient lives in this profile (ISMI).

Table 13.1: Sex and Level of Discrimination

Sl. No	*Sex*	*Level of Discrimination Experience*			*Total*
		Low	*Moderate*	*High*	
1.	Male	80(78.4)(27.7)	35(66.0)(12.1)	95(70.9)(32.9)	210(72.7)
2.	Female	22(21.6)(7.6)	18(34.0)(6.2)	39(29.1)(13.5)	79(27.3)
Total		**102(35.3)**	**53(18.3)**	**134(46.4)**	**289(100)**

Table 13.1 shows the level of prejudice experienced by male and female MDR-TB patients. 72.7 per cent of male respondents were discriminated against, with 27.7% having a low level of discrimination, 12.1% having a moderate level of discrimination, and 32.9 per cent having a high level of discrimination. There were 27.3% of female respondents, with 7.6% having a low level of discrimination, 10.4% having a moderate level of discrimination, and 3.5% having a low level of discrimination.

Table 13.2 it can be seen that the age and level of discrimination of the respondents fall into the following groups: At the age of 18 to 30, patients with MDR tuberculosis made up 24.6% of the total population. Of this population, 8.3% had a low level of discrimination, while there was a moderate degree of discrimination among 3.8% and 12.5% of the population.

Table 13.2: Age and Level of Discrimination

Sl. No.	*Age of the Patients*	*Level of Discrimination Experience*			*Total*
		Low	*Moderate*	*High*	
1.	18 to 30 years	24(23.5)(8.3)	11(20.8)(3.8)	36(26.9)(12.5)	71(24.6)
2.	31 to 40 years	18(17.6)(6.2)	9(17.0)(3.1)	15(11.2)(5.2)	42(14.5)
3.	41 to 50 years	21(20.6)(7.3)	15(28.3)(5.2)	29(21.6)(10.0)	65(22.5)
4.	51 to 60 years	27(26.5)(9.3)	13(24.5)(4.5)	33(24.6) 11.4)	73(25.3)
5.	Above 60 years	12(11.8)(4.2)	5(9.4)(1.7)	21(15.7)(7.3)	38(13.1)
	Total	**102(35.3)**	**53(18.3)**	**134(46.4)**	**289(100)**

The proportion of people between the ages of 31 and 40 who were in the patient population was 14.5%, of whom 6.2% had a low level of discrimination, 3.1% had a moderate level of discrimination, and 5.2% had a high level of discrimination. Among those ages 41 to 50, 22.5% of the patients were in the category of having a low level of discrimination, 5.2% were in the category of having a moderate level of discrimination, and 10 per cent were in the category of having a high level of discrimination.

Among those aged 51 to 60, 25.3% of patients had a lower level of discrimination, 9.3% of patients had a moderate level of discrimination, 4.5% of patients had a high level of discrimination, and 11.4% of patients were more discriminating. Patients who were beyond the age of 60 accounted for 13.1% of the total patient population. 4.2% of those patients had high-level discrimination, while 1.7% had moderate stereotype levels, and the remaining 7.3% had higher levels of discrimination.

Among those aged 51 to 60, 25.3 per cent had a lower level of discrimination, 9.3 per cent had a moderate level of discrimination, 4.5 per cent had a high level of discrimination, and 11.4 per cent had a higher level of discrimination. Patients over the age of 60 constituted 13.1 per cent of the total patient population. 4.2 per cent of the patients experienced high-level discrimination, 1.7 per cent experienced moderate stereotype levels, and the remaining 7.3 per cent experienced higher levels of discrimination.

The age and level of discrimination among interviewees were noted. Patients who were aged 18–30 had MDR-TB were 24.6% of whom 8.3% had low levels of prejudice, and 3.8% and 12.5% had moderate levels of discrimination, respectively.

Table 13.3: Religion and Level of Discrimination

Sl. No.	*The Religion of the Patients*	*Level of Discrimination Experience*			*Total*
		Low	*Moderate*	*High*	
1.	Hindu	95(93.1)(32.9)	49(92.5)(17.0)	121(90.3)(41.9)	265(91.7)
2.	Muslim	6(5.9)(2.1)	1(1.9)(0.3)	9(6.7)(3.1)	16(5.5)
3.	Christian	1(1.0)(0.3)	3(5.7)(1.0)	4(3.0)(1.4)	8(2.8)
Total		**102(35.3)**	**53(18.3)**	**134(46.4)**	**289(100)**

Table 13.3 shows that religion is associated with the amount of discrimination in patients with MDR-TB. Seventeen per cent of Hindus were discriminated against at low levels, while the bulk of Hindus (41.9 per cent) were discriminated against highly.

There were 5.5% of patients with MDR-TB who were Muslims, of which 2,1% had low discriminating levels, which implies 0.3% had low discriminatory levels, and 3,1% had moderate discrimination. 2.8 per cent of Christians with MDR-TB were Christians. Of them, 2.1 had low levels of prejudice, 0.3% had moderate levels of discrimination, and 1% had greater levels of discrimination.

The bulk of the respondents (91.7%) were Hindu, although Hindus (41.9%) claimed increased prejudice against Muslims and Christians. Approximately 5.5% of the population was determined to be Muslims. Of them, around 3.1 per cent reported "strong prejudice" and the remaining 2.8 per cent reported high discrimination.

Table 13.4: Education and Level of Discrimination

Sl. No.	*Education*	*Level of Discrimination Experience*			*Total*
		Low	*Moderate*	*High*	
1.	Illiterate	7(6.9)(2.4)	2(3.8)(0.7)	12(9.0)(4.2)	21(7.3)
2.	Primary level	18(17.6)(6.2)	11(20.8)(3.8)	31(23.1)(10.7)	60(20.8)
3.	High School	36(35.3)(12.5)	19(35.8)(6.6)	41(30.6)(14.2)	96(33.2)

Sl. No.	*Education*	*Level of Discrimination Experience*			*Total*
		Low	*Moderate*	*High*	
4.	Higher Secondary	20(19.6)(6.9)	9(17.0)(3.1)	28(20.9)(9.7)	57(19.7)
5.	Under graduation	11(10.8)(3.8)	6(11.3)(2.1)	12(9.0)(4.2)	29(10.0)
6.	Post graduation	7(6.9)(2.4)	5(9.4)(1.7)	6(4.5)(2.1)	18(6.2)
7.	Others	3(2.9)(1.0)	1(1.9)(0.3)	4(3.0)(1.4)	8(2.8)
	Total	**102(35.3)**	**53(18.3)**	**134(46.4)**	**289(100)**

The education and level of discrimination are shown in the data above in Table 13.4 Of these patients, 7.3 per cent were illiterate and 2,4 per cent had low discrimination. 0.7 per cent of them had a moderate level of discrimination and 4.2% of them were noted as having a higher level of discrimination.

Among patients who had finished primary school (5th class), 20.8% were qualified, with 6.2% falling into the "low level of discrimination" category, and 3.8% into the "moderate level of discrimination" group and 10.7 per cent of them had a high level of discrimination.

High school graduates represented 33.2% of the eligible patients. Of these, 12.5% had a low level of discrimination, whereas 6.6% had a moderate level of discrimination. Of those, 14.2% had a higher level of discrimination.

In this group, 3.1% of the patients had a low level of discrimination, 3.1% had a moderate level of discrimination, and 9.7% had a higher level of discrimination.1 in 10 respondents had graduated, of which 3.8% had a moderate level of discrimination, and 4.2% had a low level of discrimination. Among the people surveyed who studied for a degree were 10%, among whom 3.8% had a low level of prejudice. 2,1% suffered from moderate discrimination, and 4.2% had a higher level of discrimination.

The percentage of patients who completed their studies beyond a postgraduate level was 6.2%, with 2.4% of them having mild prejudice, 1.7% of them having moderate prejudice, and 2.1% of them having high prejudice.

Specifically, of the total patients who took the exam, those who studied another educational credential showed 2.8% favouritism, while among them, 0.3% had a low level of discrimination, 0.3% had a moderate level of discrimination, and 1.4% had a high degree of prejudice.

Table 13.5: Marital Status and Level of Discrimination

Sl. No.	*Marital Status*	*Level of Discrimination Experience*			*Total*
		Low	*Moderate*	*High*	
1.	Unmarried	20(19.6)(6.9)	10(18.9)(3.5)	30(22.4)(10.4)	60(20.8)
2.	Married	72(70.6)(24.9)	40(75.5)(13.8)	88(65.7)(30.4)	200(69.2)
3.	Separated	4(3.9)(1.4)	1(1.9)(0.3)	6(4.5)(2.1)	11(3.8)
4.	Widow/er	6(5.9)(2.1)	2(3.8)(0.7)	10(7.5)(3.5)	18(6.2)
	Total	**102(35.3)**	**53(18.3)**	**134(46.4)**	**289(100)**

The marital status of respondents and the level of discrimination against MDR-TB are given in Table 13.5. 20.8% of the respondents were unmarried, 6.9% experienced low levels of prejudice, 3.5% experienced moderate discrimination, and 10.4% enjoyed higher levels of discrimination.

69.2% of patients were married and 29.9% had low levels of discrimination, 13.8% had moderate levels of discrimination and 30.4% experienced greater levels of discrimination.3.8% of MDR-TB patients were separated from their spouse, 1.4% had low levels of discrimination, 0.3% had moderate discrimination, and 2.1% had higher levels of discrimination.

6.2% of the patients were widows or widows, and 2,1% of those suffered mild prejudice. 0.7 per cent had moderate degrees of discrimination, while 3.5 per cent had greater levels of discrimination.

Table 13.6: Type of Family and Level of Discrimination

Sl. No.	*Type of Family*	*Level of Discrimination Experience*			*Total*
		Low	*Moderate*	*High*	
1.	Joint Family	7(6.9)(2.4)	11(20.8)(3.8)	15(11.2)(5.2)	33(11.4)
2.	Nuclear Family	88(86.3)(30.4)	41(77.4)(14.2)	111(82.8)(38.4)	240(83.0)

Sl. No.	Type of Family	Level of Discrimination Experience			Total
		Low	Moderate	High	
3.	Not Applicable	7(6.9)(2.4)	1(1.9)(0.3)	8(6.0)(2.8)	16(5.5)
	Total	**102(35.3)**	**53(18.3)**	**134(46.4)**	**289(100)**

The family type and the amount of discrimination of MDR-TB patients are presented in Table 13.6. In joint households, patients accounted for 11.4% of the population and 2.4% of them experienced moderate prejudice. 3.8% of them reported moderate prejudice, while 5.2% were discriminated against highly.

Patients in nuclear families accounted for 83.0% of the population, 30.4% of whom had low levels of prejudice, 14.2% had moderate levels of discrimination and 38.4% had a high degree of discrimination. Among those living independently - not in a single-family or in a nuclear family - 5.5% reported low levels of discrimination, 2.4% reported moderate levels of discrimination, and 2.8% reported severe levels of prejudice.

Table 13.7: Number of Family Members and Level of Discrimination

Sl. No.	Number of Family Members	Level of Discrimination Experience			Total
		Low	Moderate	High	
1.	One	5(4.9)(1.7)	2(3.8)(0.7)	11(8.2)(3.8)	18(6.2)
2.	Two	38(37.3)(13.1)	18(34.0)(6.2)	55(41.0)(19.0)	111(38.4)
3.	3 to 5	52(51.0)(18.0)	31(58.5)(10.7)	64(47.8)(22.1)	147(50.9)
4.	Above 5	7(6.9)(2.4)	2(3.8)(0.7)	4(3.0)(1.4)	13(4.5)
	Total	**102(35.3)**	**53(18.3)**	**134(46.4)**	**289(100)**

The number of family members and the degree of discrimination among MDR-TB patients is shown in Table 13.7. Patients with one family member accounted for 6.2% of the total, with low levels of prejudice in 1.7%, moderate discrimination in 0.7%, low discrimination in 3.8%.

Patients with two family members were 38,4%, 13,1% with a low degree of discrimination, 6,2% with a moderate level of prejudice, and 19% with a high level of discrimination.

Patients with 3 to 5 members of the family make up 50.9% of the population; 18% have had low levels of prejudice, 10.7% have had modest levels of discrimination and 22.1% have suffered low levels of discrimination.

Patients in their families with more than five members accounted for 4.5% of the total, with mild prejudice at 2.4%, moderate discrimination at 0.7% and greater discrimination at 1.4%.

Table 13.8: Employment Status and Level of Discrimination

Sl. No.	*Employment Status*	*Level of Discrimination Experience*			*Total*
		Low	*Moderate*	*High*	
1.	Employed	48(47.1)(16.6)	23(43.4)(8.0)	57(42.5)(19.7)	128(44.3)
2.	Unemployed	37(36.3)(12.8)	23(43.4)(8.0)	50(37.3)(17.3)	110(38.1)
3.	Student	12(11.8)(4.2)	3(5.7)(1.0)	15(11.2)(5.2)	30(10.4)
4.	Housewife	5(4.9)(1.7)	4(7.5)(1.4)	12(9.0)(4.2)	21(7.3)
Total		**102(35.3)**	**53(18.3)**	**134(46.4)**	**289(100)**

The employment status and level of discrimination of MDR-TB patients by workplace are described in Table 13.8. Patients employed accounted for 44.3% of all, with a low level of prejudice of 16.6%, a modest level of discrimination of 8% and a severe level of discrimination of 19.7%.

Patients who have been jobless account for 38.1% of the population, 12.8% for low-level discrimination, 8% for moderate discrimination, and 17.3% for high-level prejudice.

Patients who were students accounted for 10.4% of the population, 4.2% for mild discrimination, 1% for moderate discrimination, and 5.2% for high-level discrimination.

Housewives represent 7.3% of the total. 1.7% of them suffer from low levels of prejudice, 1.4% of them suffer from moderate discrimination and 4.2% suffer from high levels of discrimination.

According to the statistics above, MDR-TB patients (44.3%) had significant levels of discrimination, whereas those who were unemployed (27.3%) were highly discriminated against 17.3

Table 13.9: Type of Employment and Level of Discrimination

Sl. No.	*Type of Employment*	*Level of Discrimination Experience*			*Total*
		Low	*Moderate*	*High*	
1.	Government	7(6.9)(2.4)	2(3.8)(0.7)	8(6.0)(2.8)	17(5.9)
2.	Private	10(9.8)(3.5)	4(7.5)(1.4)	9(6.7)(3.1)	23(8.0)
3.	Labour/Daily wages	29(28.4)(10.0)	15(28.3)(5.2)	29(21.6)(10.0)	73(25.3)
4.	Self Employed	2(2.0)(0.7)	2(3.8)(0.7)	11(8.2)(3.8)	15(5.2)
5.	Not Applicable	54(52.9)(18.7)	30(56.6)(10.4)	77(57.5)(26.6)	161(55.7)
Total		**102(35.3)**	**53(18.3)**	**134(46.4)**	**289(100)**

Table 13.9 illustrates the kind of work and level of discrimination of respondents in respect of the discrimination against MDR-TB. Of the respondents, 5.9% worked in government, 2.4% had mild prejudice, 0.7% had moderate discrimination and 2.8% had a high degree of discrimination. Private patients represented 8 per cent of the total, 3.5 per cent experienced mild discrimination, 1.4 per cent experienced moderate discrimination and 3.1 per cent were discriminated against at high levels.

Of MDR-TB patients, 25.3% worked as a worker/daily employee, 10% had a low level of discrimination and 5.2% had a moderate level of discrimination, and 10% had a high level of discrimination. Patients self-employed represented 5.2% of the total and 0.7% had mild to high levels of discrimination. In this category, 3.8% of respondents were discriminated against at low levels. More than half of respondents (55.7 per cent) were not qualified for jobs, according to the table above. There was a low degree of prejudice in 18,7%, a moderate level of discrimination in 10,4% and a high level of discrimination in 26,6%.

Table 13.10: Monthly Income and Level of Discrimination

Sl. No.	*Monthly Income*	*Level of Discrimination Experience*			*Total*
		Low	*Moderate*	*High*	
1.	Up to 5000	20(19.6)(6.9)	11(20.8)(3.8)	23(17.2)(8.0)	54(18.7)
2.	5001 to 10000	14(13.7)(4.8)	7(13.2)(2.4)	23(17.2)(8.0)	44(15.2)

Sl. No.	*Monthly Income*	*Level of Discrimination Experience*			*Total*
		Low	*Moderate*	*High*	
3.	above 10000	13(12.7)(4.5)	5(9.4)(1.7)	11(8.2)(3.8)	29(10.0)
4.	Not Applicable	55(53.9)(19.0)	30(56.6)(10.4)	77(57.5)(26.6)	162(56.1)
Total		**102(35.3)**	**53(18.3)**	**134(46.4)**	**289(100)**

Table 13.10 shows the association between MDR-TB patients' income levels and their level of discrimination. Patients with a monthly income of up to Rs. 5000/-had a low level of discrimination (18.7%), a moderate level of discrimination (3.8%), and a low level of discrimination (8%).

Patients with monthly incomes ranging from Rs. 5001/- to Rs. 10000/-made up 15.2 per cent of the total, with 4.8% experiencing low-level discrimination, 2.4% experiencing moderate level discrimination, and 8% experiencing low-level discrimination. The respondents who had a monthly salary of more than Rs. 10,000/were 10%, and 4.5% had a low level of discrimination, 1.7% had a moderate level of discrimination, and 38% had a high level of discrimination.

According to the table, more than half of the respondents (56.1 per cent) had no income, implying that they were not eligible for any income. Nineteen per cent of the patients reported low discrimination, whereas 10.4 per cent experienced moderate discrimination. A high level of prejudice was experienced by 26.6 per cent of them.

According to the above table, more than half of the respondents (56.1%) were not eligible for any source of income. In this category, 19% had a low level of discrimination, 10.4% had a moderate level of discrimination, and 26.6% had a high level of discrimination.

Table 13.11: Length of Treatment and Level of Discrimination

Sl. No.	*Length of Treatment*	*Level of Discrimination Experience*			*Total*
		Low	*Moderate*	*High*	
1.	Less than 1 year	35(34.3)(12.1)	24(45.3)(8.3)	58(43.3)(20.1)	117(40.5)
2.	1 to 2 years	67(65.7)(23.2)	29(54.7)(10.0)	76(56.7)(26.3)	172(59.5)
Total		**102(35.3)**	**53(18.3)**	**134(46.4)**	**289(100)**

The above Table 13.11 shows the length of MDR-TB treatment and the amount of discrimination faced by MDR-TB patients. Patients who had been on MDR-TB medication for less than a year represented 40.5 per cent of the total; 12.1% reported evidence of low-level discrimination, 8.3% had evidence of moderate level discrimination, and 20.1% had evidence of high-level discrimination. Patients who were on MDR-TB medication for one to two years (59.5%) had a low level of discrimination, 10% had a moderate level of discrimination, and 26.3 had a high level of discrimination.

Table 13.12: Family Support and Level of Discrimination

Sl. No.	*Family Support*	*Level of Discrimination Experience*			*Total*
		Low	*Moderate*	*High*	
1.	Yes	21(20.6)(7.3)	12(22.6)(4.2)	38(28.4)(13.1)	71(24.6)
2.	No	81(79.4)(28.0)	41(77.4)(14.2)	96(71.6)(33.2)	218(75.4)
Total		**102(35.3)**	**53(18.3)**	**134(46.4)**	**289(100)**

The above Table 13.12 shows family member support throughout illness as well as the level of discrimination experienced by MDR-TB patients. The patients on treatment for MDR-TB illness, family member support were (24.6 per cent), of whom 7.3 per cent had evidence of low-level discrimination, 4.2 per cent had evidence of moderate level discrimination, and 13.1 per cent had evidence of low-level discrimination.

The majority 75.4 per cent of patients receiving MDR-TB treatment reported that there is no family member support throughout the illness of the MDR-TB patients, 28 per cent of whom had evidence of low-level discrimination, 14.2 per cent of whom had evidence of moderate level discrimination, and 33.2 per cent of whom had evidence of high-level discrimination.

It was discovered that the vast majority of respondents, three-fourths (75.4 per cent), reported no family member support during the illness of MDR-TB patients, while one-fourth (24.6 per cent) reported no support throughout the illness.

Table 13.13: Feeling of Isolation and Level of Discrimination

Sl. No.	*Feeling of Isolation*	*Level of Discrimination Experience*			*Total*
		Low	*Moderate*	*High*	
1.	Yes	71(69.6)(24.6)	26(49.1)(9.0)	81(60.4)(28.0)	178(61.6)
2.	No	31(30.4)(10.7)	27(50.9)(9.3)	53(39.6)(18.3)	111(38.4)
Total		**102(35.3)**	**53(18.3)**	**134(46.4)**	**289(100)**

Table 13.13 shows the experience of isolation and the amount of discrimination. These patients' relatives experience discrimination, as shown by a lack of empathy and connection in their table of findings.

To assess this association, it was found out that the majority of respondents (61.6%) reported being isolated from their family members due to MDR-TB. Twenty-eight per cent of participants reported experiencing high levels of discrimination as a result of their MDR-TB illness, while 24.6 per cent reported experiencing low types of discrimination.

It was found that the vast majority of respondents (61.6 per cent) reported being isolated and discriminated against by their family members owing to MDR-TB, whereas 38.4 per cent of respondents reported not being isolated or discriminated against by their family members.

Table 13.14: Isolation from Family Members and Level of Discrimination

Chi-Square Test

H_0: There is no association between feeling of isolation from family members and level of discrimination.

Chi-Square Tests			
	Value	***df***	***Asymp. Sig.(2-sided)***
Pearson Chi-Square	6.365[a]	2	.041
Likelihood Ratio	6.353	2	.042
Linear-by-Linear Association	1.708	1	.191
No. of Valid Cases	289		

a. 0 cells (0.0%) have an expected count less than 5. The minimum expected count is 20.36.

Table 13.14 shows that the association between feeling of isolation from family members and level of discrimination. The Chi-Square Test has proved that there is no association between feeling of isolation from family members and level of discrimination

Table 13.15: Taking Daily Food with Family Members and Level of Discrimination

Sl. No.	*Daily Food Intake with a Family Member*	*Level of Discrimination Experience*			*Total*
		Low	*Moderate*	*High*	
1.	Yes	47(46.1)(16.3)	27(50.9)(9.3)	61(45.5)(21.1)	135(46.7)
2.	No	55(53.9)(19.0)	26(49.1)(9.0)	73(54.5)(25.3)	154(53.3)
	Total	**102(35.3)**	**53(18.3)**	**134(46.4)**	**289(100)**

Table 13.15 shows whether the patient takes the daily food along with the family members or the patient is being provided food separately due to TB illness. It is noticed that 46.7 per cent of the MDR-TB patients take the daily food along with their family members, among these patients 16.3 per cent of them had a low level of discrimination were from North Chennai, (12.5%) from East Chennai, 10.7 per cent of the patients were from Central Chennai, 6.2 per cent of the patients were from West Chennai, and 2.4 per cent from south Chennai.

53.3 per cent of the respondents shared that they were being provided food separately due to TB illness, among them (15.9%) patients were from North Chennai, 14.2 per cent from East Chennai, (9.7%) from Central Chennai, (6.2%) from West Chennai and 7.3 per cent of the patients belonged to South Chennai.

It is noticed that 46.7 per cent of the MDR-TB patients take the daily food along with their family members and 53.31 per cent of the respondents shared that they were being provided food separately due to TB illness.

The sex and level of stigma resistance among male and female MDR-TB patients are shown in Table No: 13.16. Men suffer a higher level of stigma with regards to MDR-TB. Specifically, 72.7% of the men felt discriminated against by MDR-TB. However, 28.4% had a low level of stigma resistance, 14.2% had a moderate level of stigma resistance, and 30.1% had a high level of stigma resistance. 27,3% of female respondents indicated that they had a low level of stigma resistance; 11.8% noted that they had a low level of stigma resistance; 5.9% noted that they had a moderate level of stigma resistance, and 9.7% of respondents indicated that they had a high level of stigma resistance.

Table 13.16: Sex and Level of Stigma Resistance

Sl. No.	*Sex*	*Level of Stigma Resistance*			*Total*
		Low	*Moderate*	*High*	
1.	Male	82(70.7)(28.4)	41(70.7)(14.2)	87(75.7)(30.1)	210(72.7)
2.	Female	34(29.3)(11.8)	17(29.3)(5.9)	28(24.3)(9.7)	79(27.3)
Total		**116(40.1)**	**58(20.1)**	**115(39.8)**	**289(100)**

Table 13.17: Age and Level of Stigma Resistance

Sl. No.	*Age of the Patients*	*Level of Stigma Resistance*			*Total*
		Low	*Moderate*	*High*	
1.	18 to 30 years	28(24.1)(9.7)	11(19.0)(3.8)	32(27.8)(11.1)	71(24.6)
2.	30 to 40 years	19(16.4)(6.6)	4(6.9)(1.4)	19(16.5)(6.6)	42(14.5)
3.	41 to 50 Years	28(24.1)(9.7)	12(20.7)(4.2)	25(21.7)(8.7)	65(22.5)
4.	51 to 60 years	29(25.0)(10.0)	18(31.0)(6.2)	26(22.6)(9.0)	73(25.3)
5.	Above 60 years	12(10.3)(4.2)	13(22.4)(4.5)	13(11.3)(4.5)	38(13.1)
Total		**116(40.1)**	**58(20.1)**	**115(39.8)**	**289(100)**

From the data in Table 13.17, it can be seen that respondents fall into the following age and stigma resistance categories: About 24.6% of the total population was made up of patients with multidrug-resistant tuberculosis at the age of 18 to 30. 9.7% of this population had low stigma resistance, while 3.8% of the population had moderate stigma resistance and 11.1% of the population had a high level of stigma resistance. This proportion of the population between the ages of 31 and 40 was 14.5%, with 6.6% having a low and higher level of stigma resistance, while 1.4% having a moderate level of stigma resistance.

Over the age of 41 to 50, nearly 22.5% of the patients fell into this category. Among them, a low level of stigma resistance noted was 9.7. Of the rest, 4.2% fell into the moderate stigma resistance category and 8.7% belonged to the high stigma resistance category. Those patients who are between the ages of 51 and 60 comprise 25.3% of the total group. 9.7 per cent of the patients expressed a low level of stigma resistance, 6.2% reported a moderate level of stigma resistance, and 9% expressed a high level of stigma resistance.

13.1% of the patient population was over the age of 60. 4.2 per cent of patients had a low level of stigma resistance, 4.5 per cent had a moderate level of stigma resistance, and also a higher level of stigma resistance.

Stigma resistance was observed to be associated with age and stage of development. Of the 24.6% of patients with MDR-TB who were between the ages of 18 and 30, 9.7% were considered to have low stigma resistance, while 3.8% and 11.1% were moderate. Among adults aged 51 to 60, 25.3% had suffered a low level of stigma, 6.2% had experienced a moderate level of stigma, and 9% had experienced high stigma.

Table 13.18: Religion and Level of Stigma Resistance

Sl. No.	*The Religion of the Patients*	*Level of Stigma Resistance*			*Total*
		Low	*Moderate*	*High*	
1.	Hindu	108(93.1)(37.4)	52(89.7)18.0)	105(91.30)(36.3)	265(91.7)
2.	Muslim	4(3.4)(1.4)	4(6.9)(1.4)	8(7.0)(2.8)	16(5.5)
3.	Christian	4(3.4)(1.4)	2(3.4)(0.7)	2(1.7)(0.7)	8(2.8)
	Total	**116(40.1)**	**58(20.1)**	**115(39.8)**	**289(100)**

Table 13.18 illustrates that religion is linked to TB patients' stigma resistance. Hinduism has about 91.7% of the patients as participants. Majority The incidence of stigma resistance was higher in 37.4% of Hindus, while moderate and high stigma resistance occurred at lower percentages in 18% and 36.3%, respectively.

Nearly 5% of the MDR-TB patients identified as Muslims, with about 1.4% fulfilling the requirements for having low or moderate levels of stigma resistance, and about 2.8% revealed high levels of stigma resistance. And within the Christian religion, 2.8% of patients had MDR tuberculosis. Stigma resistance was found at the low levels of 1.4% of the respondents; a percentage of 0.7% of the participants had high or moderate levels of stigma resistance.

More than nine out of ten respondents (91.7%) were Hindus, with nearly 36% of those identified with that religion reporting higher levels of stigma resistance as compared to Muslims and Christians. A survey revealed that Muslims comprised about 5.5% of the population. About 2.8 per cent of the population reported having "high levels of stigma resistance" and Christians were found to be about 2.8% of the population. Of those, about 0.7% reported experiencing "high levels of stigma resistance."

Table 13.19: Education and Level of Stigma Resistance

Sl. No.	*Education*	*Level of Stigma Resistance*			*Total*
		Low	*Moderate*	*High*	
1.	Illiterate	5(4.3)(1.7)	8(13.8)(2.8)	8(7.0)(2.8)	21(7.3)
2.	Primary level	21(18.1)(7.3)	12(20.7)(4.2)	27(23.5)(9.3)	60(19.7)
3.	High School	46(39.7)(15.9)	16(27.6)(5.5)	34(29.6)(11.8)	96(33.2)
4.	Higher Secondary	19(16.4)(6.6)	13(22.4)(4.5)	25(21.7)(8.7)	57(19.7)
5.	Under graduation	10(8.6)(3.5)	2(3.4)(0.7)	17(14.8)(5.9)	29(10.0)
6.	Post graduation	12(10.3)(4.2)	4(6.9)(1.4)	2(1.7)(0.7)	18(6.2)
7.	Others	3(2.6)(1.0)	3(5.2)(1.0)	2(1.7)(0.7)	8(2.8)
Total		**116(40.1)**	**58(20.1)**	**115(39.8)**	**289(100)**

The data in Table 13.19 shows the level of education and stigma resistance. 7.3 per cent of the patients were illiterate, and 1.7 per cent had a low level of stigma resistance. Stigma resistance was found to be moderate and high amongst 2.8 per cent of them.

20.8 per cent of patients who had completed primary education (5th grade) were eligible, with 7.3 per cent having a "low degree of stigma resistance" and 4,2 per cent having a "moderate level of stigma resistance." 9.3% of them exhibited a high level of stigma resistance, according to the book.33.2 per cent of those who were eligible were in high school. 15.9% of those surveyed showed a low level of stigma resistance, while 5.5 per cent had a moderate level. 11.8 per cent of individuals surveyed reported a greater level of stigma resistance.

19.7% of the patients were in the upper secondary category, with 6.6 per cent having a low level of stigma resistance, 4,5 per cent having a moderate level of stigma resistance, and 8.7% have a higher degree of stigma resistance.10% of those surveyed who were booking for a degree had a low level of stigma resistance, whereas 3.5 per cent had a high level of stigma. Only 0.7 per cent had a moderate level of stigma resistance, whereas 5.9 per cent had high stigma resistance.

Patients who completed their studies at the postgraduate level accounted for 6.2 per cent of the total, with 4.2 per cent having mild stigma resistance, 1.4 per cent having severe stigma resistance, and 0.7 per cent having high stigma resistance. Patients who studied another educational credential showed a 2.8 per cent preference, with one per cent having a low to moderate level of stigma resistance and 0.7 per cent having a high level of stigma resistance among those who took the exam.

The percentage of people who finished high school was found to be 33.2 per cent. 15.9% of those surveyed showed a low level of stigma resistance, while 5.5 per cent had a moderate level. 11.8 per cent of individuals surveyed had a higher level of stigma resistance.

Table 13.20: Marital Status and Level of Stigma Resistance

Sl. No.	*Marital Status*	*Level of Stigma Resistance*			*Total*
		Low	*Moderate*	*High*	
1.	Unmarried	24(20.7)(8.3)	8(13.8)(2.8)	28(24.3)(9.7)	60(20.8)
2.	Married	83(71.6)(28.7)	43(74.1)(14.9)	74(64.3)(25.6)	200(69.2)
3.	Separated	4(3.4)(1.4)	1(1.7)(0.3)	6(5.2)(2.1)	11(3.8)
4.	Widow/er	5(4.3)(1.7)	6(10.3)(2.1)	7(6.1)(2.4)	18(6.2)
	Total	**116(40.1)**	**58(20.1)**	**115(39.8)**	**289(100)**

MDR-TB stigma resistance levels are listed in Table 13.20. About 20.8% of participants were unmarried, and 8.3% reported low levels of stigma resistance, 2.8% reported moderate levels of stigma resistance, and 9.7% reported higher levels of stigma resistance. 69.2% of patients were married, and 28.7% had low levels of stigma resistance, 14.9 per cent had moderate levels of stigma resistance, and 25.6 per cent had high levels of stigma resistance.

More than 3.8% of patients with multi-drug resistant tuberculosis (MDR-TB) were separated from their spouse; one-and-a-half per cent reported low levels of stigma resistance, while less than three per cent reported moderate levels of stigma resistance, and 2.1% reported higher levels of stigma resistance.

Low-level stigma resistance took place for 6.2% of patients who were widows or widowers, with 1.7% falling into this category. In 2.1% of them, there was moderate resistance to stigma, while in 2.4% of them, there was higher resistance to stigma. The authors found that nearly seven in ten (69.2 per cent) of the patients were married. One-third (28.7%) of the respondents had low stigma tolerance, fourteen out of ten (14.9%) of the respondents had a tolerance for mild stigma, and one-fourth (25.6 per cent) of the respondents reported encountering increased stigma.

Table 13.21: Type of Family and Level of Stigma Resistance

Sl No.	*Type of Family*	*Level of Stigma Resistance*			*Total*
		Low	*Moderate*	*High*	
1.	Joint Family	13(11.2)(4.5)	8(13.8)(2.8)	12(10.4)(4.2)	33(11.4)
2.	Nuclear Family	97(83.6)(33.6)	48(82.8)(16.6)	95(82.6)(32.9)	240(83.1)
3.	Not Applicable	6(5.2)(2.1)	2(3.4)(0.7)	8(7.0)(2.8)	16(5.5)
Total		**116(40.1)**	**58(20.1)**	**115(39.8)**	**289(100)**

The type of family in which MDR-TB patients live and their level of stigma resistance are shown in Table 13.21. Patients who lived in joint families represented 11.4 per cent of the population, and 4.5 per cent of them experienced mild levels of stigma resistance. 2,8 per cent of them experienced moderate levels of stigma resistance, while 4.2 per cent experienced high levels of stigma resistance.

Patients who lived in nuclear families accounted for 83.0 per cent of the population, with 33.6 per cent experiencing low levels of stigma resistance, 16.6 per cent experiencing moderate levels of stigma resistance, and 32.9 per cent experiencing high levels of stigma resistance.

Among the respondents who lived separately, 5.5 per cent, neither in a joint family nor in a nuclear family, 2,1 per cent reported having low levels of stigma resistance, 0.7 per cent reported experiencing moderate levels of stigma resistance, and 2.8 per cent reported experiencing high levels of stigma resistance.

Table 13.22: Number of Family Members and Level of Stigma Resistance

Sl No.	*No. of Family Members*	*Level of Stigma Resistance*			*Total*
		Low	*Moderate*	*High*	
1.	One	5(4.3)(1.7)	6(10.3)(2.1)	7(6.1)(2.4)	18(6.2)
2.	Two	41(35.3)(14.2)	22(37.9(7.6)	48(41.7)(16.6)	111(38.4)
3.	3 to 5	62(53.4)(21.5)	27(46.6)(9.3)	58(50.4)(20.1)	147(50.9)
4.	Above 5	8(6.9)(2.8)	3(5.2)(1.0)	2(1.7)(0.7)	13(4.5)
Total		**116(40.1)**	**58(20.1)**	**115(39.8)**	**289(100)**

Table 13.22 shows the number of family members and level of stigma resistance among MDR-TB patients. Patients with one member in the family made up 6.2% of the total, with 1.7% experiencing low-level stigma resistance, 2.1% experiencing moderate level stigma resistance, and 2.4% experiencing low-level stigma resistance. The patients who had two members in their family were 38.4%, with 14.2% having a low level of stigma resistance, 7.6% having a moderate level of stigma resistance, and 16.6% having a high level of stigma resistance.

Patients with three to five family members made up 50.9 per cent of the population; 21.5 per cent experienced low levels of stigma resistance, 9.3 per cent experienced moderate levels of stigma resistance, and 20.1 per cent experienced low levels of stigma resistance. Patients with more than five members in their family accounted for 4.5% of the total, with 2.8 per cent of the respondents experiencing low-level stigma resistance, one per cent experiencing moderate level stigma resistance, and 0.7% experiencing higher-level stigma resistance.

The job status and level of stigma resistance of MDR-TB patients in the workplace are shown in Table 13.23 The employed patients accounted up 44.3 per cent of the total, with 18% having a low degree of stigma resistance, 9.7 per cent having a moderate level of stigma resistance, and 16.6 per cent having a high level of stigma resistance.

Table 13.23: Employment Status and Level of Stigma

Sl. No.	*Employment Status*	*Level of Stigma Resistance*			*Total*
		Low	*Moderate*	*High*	
1.	Employed	52(44.8)(18.0)	28(48.3)(9.7)	48(41.7)(16.6)	128(44.3)
2.	Unemployed	44(37.9)(15.2)	20(34.5)(6.9)	46(40.0)(15.9)	110(38.1)
3.	Student	12(10.3)(4.2)	4(6.9)(1.4)	14(12.2)(4.8)	30(10.4)
4.	Housewife	8(6.9)(2.8)	6(10.3)(2.1)	7(6.1)(2.4)	21(7.3)
Total		**116(40.1)**	**58(20.1)**	**115(39.8)**	**289(100)**

Unemployed patients accounted for 38.1 per cent of the population, with 15.2 per cent exhibiting low-level stigma resistance, 6.9 per cent exhibiting moderate-level stigma resistance, and 15.9 per cent exhibiting high-level stigma resistance.

Students made up 10.4 per cent of the population, with 4.2 per cent having low-level stigma resistance, 1.4 per cent having moderate-level stigma resistance, and 4.8 per cent having high-level stigma resistance.

According to the findings, MDR-TB patients who were employed (44.3 per cent) had a high level of stigma resistance, whereas unemployed patients accounted for 38.1 per cent of the population, with 15.9 per cent having a high level of stigma resistance.

Table 13.24: Type of Employment and Level of Stigma

Sl. No.	*Type of Employment*	*Level of Stigma Resistance*			*Total*
		Low	*Moderate*	*High*	
1.	Government	5(4.3)(1.7)	4(6.9)(1.4)	8(7.0)(2.8)	17(5.9)
2.	Private	9(7.8)(3.1)	6(10.3)(2.1)	223(87.0)(2.8)	238(8.0)
3.	Labour/daily wages	35(30.2)(12.1)	12(20.7)(4.2)	26(22.6)(9.0)	73(25.3)
4.	Self Employed	3(2.6)(1.0)	6(10.3)(2.1)	6(5.2)(2.1)	15(5.2)
5.	Not Applicable	64(55.2(22.1)	30(51.7)(10.4)	67(58.)(23.2)	161(55.7)
Total		**116(40.1)**	**58(20.1)**	**115(39.8)**	**289(100)**

Table 13.24 shows the respondents' employment type and level of stigma resistance concerning MDR-TB stigma resistance. 5.9 per

cent of the respondents worked in government, with 1.7 per cent having low stigma resistance, 1.4 per cent having moderate stigma resistance, and 2.8 per cent having high stigma resistance.

Patients who work in private made up 8% of the total, with 3.1% reporting low levels of stigma resistance, 2.1 per cent experiencing moderate levels of stigma resistance, and 2.8% experiencing high levels of stigma resistance. Among MDR-TB patients, 25.3 per cent worked as labourers/daily wage earners, with 12.1 per cent having low stigma resistance, 4.2 per cent having moderate stigma resistance, and 9 per cent having high stigma resistance.

Patients who worked for themselves made up 5.2 per cent of the total, with one per cent having modest levels of stigma resistance. 2.1 per cent of responders in this group reported moderate to high levels of stigma resistance. More than half of the respondents (55.7 per cent) were ineligible for work, according to the data. In this category, 22.1 per cent had low stigma resistance, 10.4 per cent had moderate stigma resistance, and 23.2 per cent had high stigma resistance.

Table 13.25: Monthly Income and Level of Stigma

Sl. No.	*Monthly Income*	*Level of Stigma Resistance*			*Total*
		Low	*Moderate*	*High*	
1.	Up to 5000	22(19.0)(7.6)	12(20.7)(4.2)	20(17.4)(6.9)	54(18.7)
2.	5001 to 10000	19(16.4)(6.6)	11(19.0)(3.8)	14(12.2)(4.8)	44(15.2)
3.	above 10000	11(9.5)(3.8)	5(8.6)(1.7)	13(11.3)(4.5)	29(10.0)
4.	Not Applicable	64(55.2)(22.1)	30(51.7)(10.4)	68(59.1)(23.5)	162(56.1)
Total		**116(40.1)**	**58(20.1)**	**115(39.8)**	**289(100)**

The link between the income level and stigma resistance of the MDR-TB patients in Table 13.25 is shown. Patients with a monthly income of up to Rs. 5000/-, 7.6% of patients showed low resistance to stigma, moderate resilience to stigma (4.2%), and low resistance to stigma (6.9%). The monthly income range for patients ranges from Rs 5001/- to Rs 10000/-amounted to 15,2%, with 6.6% having low resistance to stigma, 3,8% with a moderate degree of stigma and 4,8% with a low level of resistance to stigma.

Those who had a monthly wage of more than Rs. 10.000/10% had low resistance to stigma, 1,7% had a modest resistance to stigma and 4,5% had a high degree of resistance to stigma. Those who earned more than Rs. 10 000 a month had 10%, while stigma resistance was little at 3.8%, moderate stigma resistance was low at 1.7% and stigma resistance was strong at 4.5%.

The chart states that over half (56.1 per cent) of respondents did not have revenue, meaning they were not eligible for income. 22.1% of patients reported resistance to stigma, while 10.4% had moderate resistance to stigma. 23.5 per cent had a high level of stigma resistance.

Table 13.26: Length of Treatment and Level of Stigma

Sl No.	*Length of Treatment*	*Level of Stigma Resistance*			*Total*
		Low	*Moderate*	*High*	
1.	Less than 1 year	46(39.7)(15.9)	23(39.7)(8.0)	48(41.7)(16.6)	117(40.5)
2.	1 to 2 years	70(60.3)(24.2)	35(60.3)(12.1)	67(58.3)(23.2)	172(59.5)
	Total	**116(40.1)**	**58(20.1)**	**115(39.8)**	**289(100)**

The above Table 13.26 shows the length of MDR-TB treatment and the amount of stigma resistance faced by MDR-TB patients. Patients who had been on MDR-TB medication for less than a year represented 40.5 per cent of the total; 15.9% reported evidence of low-level stigma resistance, 8.0% had evidence of moderate level stigma resistance, and 16.6% had evidence of high-level stigma resistance.

Patients who were on MDR-TB medication for one to two years were 59.5%). 24.2 per cent had a low level of stigma resistance, 12.1% had a moderate level of stigma resistance, and 23.2 per cent had a high level of stigma resistance.

The below Table 13.27 shows family member support throughout illness as well as the level of stigma resistance experienced by MDR-TB patients. For the patients on treatment for MDR-TB illness, family member support was (24.6 per cent), of whom ten per cent had evidence. 4.8 per cent had evidence of moderate level stigma resistance, and 9.7 per cent had evidence of high-level stigma resistance.

Table 13.27: Family Support and Level of Stigma

Sl. No.	*Family Member Support During the Illness*	*Level of Stigma Resistance*			*Total*
		Low	*Moderate*	*High*	
1.	Yes	29(25.0)(10.0)	14(24.1)(4.8)	28(24.3)(9.7)	71(24.6)
2.	No	87(75.0)(30.1)	44(75.9)(15.2)	87(75.7)(30.1)	218(75.4)
	Total	**116(40.1)**	**58(20.1)**	**115(39.8)**	**289(100)**

The majority 75.4 per cent of patients receiving MDR-TB treatment reported that there was no family member support throughout the illness of the MDR-TB patients, 30.1 per cent of whom had evidence of low-level stigma resistance, 15.2 per cent of whom had evidence of moderate level stigma resistance, and 30.1 per cent of whom had evidence of high-level stigma resistance. It was found that the vast majority of respondents, three fourths (75.4 per cent) reported that there was no family member support during the sickness of MDR-TB patients, as well as one third (30.1 per cent) evidence of high-level stigma resistance.

Table 13.28: Feeling of Isolation and Level of Stigma

Sl No.	*Feeling of Isolation*	*Level of Stigma Resistance*			*Total*
		Low	*Moderate*	*High*	
1.	Yes	65(56.0)(22.5)	35(60.3)(12.1)	78(67.8)(27.0)	178(61.6)
2.	No	51(44.0)(17.6)	23(39.7)(8.0)	37(32.2)(12.8)	111(38.4)
	Total	**116(40.1)**	**58(20.1)**	**115(39.8)**	**289(100)**

Table 13.28 shows the experience of isolation as well as the level of stigma resistance. The relatives of these patients show stigma resistance, as evidenced by a lack of empathy and connection in their table of results. To assess this association, it was discovered that the majority of respondents (61.6 per cent) reported being isolated from their family members due to MDR-TB. As a result of their MDR-TB condition, 22.5 per cent of participants reported a low level of stigma resistance, 12.1 per cent had a moderate level of stigma resistance, and

27% showed indications of high-level stigma resistance. It was found that the vast majority of respondents (61.6 per cent) reported being isolated and discriminated against by their family members owing to MDR-TB, whereas 38.4 per cent of respondents reported not being isolated or discriminated against by their family members.

Conclusion

The age and education level of the MDR-TB patients were associated with the presence of a strong family support system. With regard to family support, there was no correlation between age and education in the MDR-TB patients. The association between the monthly income of MDR tuberculosis patients and the level of family assistance was found to be related.

It was found that MDR-TB patients who have taken previous therapy for TB are strongly connected to their family support. In addition, it was discovered that the duration of TB disease of MDR-TB patients was significantly linked to the level of family assistance provided to them.

There is a considerable relationship between the cost of private TB treatment and the amount of family support provided to the MDR-TB patient. This means that it has also been found that there is no connection between the duration of the TB problem and the level of family support for patients who have extensively drug-resistant TB.

Chapter 14

MDR-TB Research: Qualitative Approach

This section includes qualitative data analysis of 5 Focus Group Discussions (FGDs) and a presentation of the findings. The focus group discussions were based on the study objectives and findings, which were highlighted.

Background of the FGD Participants

The MDR-TB patients who are taking treatment for more than 6 months and above 18 years of age have participated in the FGD. The patients who had come for treatment to the Government TB RNTCP/NTEP unit were interviewed.

The Focus of FGD and Sampling

Five focus group discussions (FGD) were conducted using the FGD interview guide, one in each health district in Chennai for this academic research. To study the support systems and overall health condition of patients to comprehend and triangulate with Quantitative Research techniques. With the consent of the authorities, the authors used MDR-TB patients gathered at the T.B unit in the districts to perform the FGD with them.

1. *Focus Group Discussion—North Chennai*

Venue: Elango Nagar TB Unit.

No of participants: 9 (7 Men and 2 Women)

The focus group discussion was conducted at Elango Nagar TB Unit in North Chennai health district between 10.30 am and 11.45 am. 9 MDR-TB patients participated in the discussion. The participants were homogenous and seven of them were male and two of them were female. The age group of the patients was 30 to 55 years old. The session lasted 1.15 minutes.

The discussion was based on the objectives of the study, viz., general health status and well-being, stigma, their family support, their treatment and the available support systems for MDR-TB patients were discussed.

The overall findings of the FGD came out with the following response:

- According to the MDR-TB patients, the majority of them were not satisfied with their health conditions due to MDR-TB. The majority of them lived in the poor physical condition and from poor families. They shared that they were not in a position to accept their body appearance because of MDR-TB. The MDR-TB patients were mostly from poor socioeconomic status and did not have enough money to meet their needs. They also shared that the personal relationships within the family are good but outside the family are poor.
- The FGD also revealed that most young people who had lost their sleep, especially the female group members, were the ones who had mostly lost their sleep worrying about MDR-TB and they were feeling unhappy and not enjoying their day-to-day activities and losing confidence.
- The FGD revealed that most of the young patients were those who were disappointed, embarrassed, isolated because of their physical appearance and kept distant from their neighbours and friends/relatives.
- The other reason gathered was that the majority of the patients received day-to-day support from their family members during the MDR-TB illness. The majority of them shared that they were not isolated by their family because of MDR-TB.
- It was also observed that most of the group members had taken previous TB treatment. Among them, one person shared that he had not taken TB treatment from private sources and the remaining patients shared that they had spent more money on TB treatment before going to the government health facility.

- Many respondents shared that they have received free treatment and diagnostic support from government health facilities. The group also revealed that there was no or negligible support from associations or NGO's for this illness. Among the group, very few members shared that they had received support from health volunteers/ASHA and DoT providers for this illness.

2. *Focus Group Discussion—East Chennai*

Venue: TPMF Thantahi Periyar TB unit-Chellappa street, Pursaiwalkam

The number of participants: 10 (6 men and 4 women).

The FGD was conducted at TPMF (Thantahi Periyar TB unit-Chellappa Street, Pursaiwalkam TB unit in East Chennai Health District. The discussion lasted from 11.00 am to 12.45 Noon. Six men and four women, altogether 10 participants, joined the FGD. The participants were between the age groups of 20 years and 50 years. The FGD was divided into two sessions; the first session was for 45 minutes; the second session was for 45 minutes with a break of 15 minutes. The FGD focused on the issues related to general health status and well-being, stigma, patients' family support, treatment and available support systems for them.

The focus group discussion brought out the following outcomes:

- Most of the patients shared that they were not in a position to accept their body appearance caused by TB. The group members mostly belonged to poor socioeconomic status and did not have enough money to meet their daily needs. They also shared that the personal relationships in the family were good, but their relationships with others outside the family were poor.
- The discussion brought out that most young people, due to worry, have lost their sleep, especially the female participants, who are worried about the disease. They were feeling unhappy and not enjoying their day-to-day activities and felt that they were losing confidence.
- Most of the participants shared that they were disappointed, embarrassed, isolated because of their physical appearance and kept aloof from their neighbours and friends/relatives.

- Group members also shared that they received day-to-day support from their family members during this illness. Except for one participant, all of them shared that they were not isolated by their family members due to this illness.
- It was also noted that most of the participants had taken TB treatment earlier. Among them, almost all of them had taken private TB treatment and, commonly, all of them had spent money on their private TB treatment before going to the government hospital for treatment.
- It was noted during the discussion that the participants received free diagnostic and treatment support from government hospitals. The group also revealed that they have not received any support from the associations or NGO's for this illness. Two participants shared that one NGO is providing him with food support during this treatment. The group members shared that they are receiving support from the volunteers/ASHA and DoT providers for this TB illness.
- FGD interview participants MDR-TB patients' names were not mentioned anywhere in this study for the confidentiality of the participants.

3. *Focus Group Discussion—Central Chennai*

Venue: Varadharajapuram-TB unit, Chennai

Number of participants: 11 (six male and 5 female)

An FGD was conducted at Varadharajapuram-TB unit, Chennai TB unit. The FGD was conducted for 1.30 minutes with a break in-between for 10 to 15 minutes from 10.30 am to 12.15 noon. There were 11 participants. Among them, there were 6 males and five female participants. The participants were in the age group between 25 years and 60 years. The authorss divided the FGD into two sessions; the first session was for 45 minutes duration and the second session was for 45 minutes with a break in between for 15 minutes for the participants.

The discussion focused on the issues related to general health status and well-being, stigma, patients' family support, treatment and available support systems for MDR-TB patients. The focus group discussion was instrumental in bringing out the problems, support and issues among the patients.

- The respondents shared that they were not satisfied with their health condition because of MDR-TB. The discussion brought out that the patients' physical living environment was bad and not a conducive habitat, and the majority of them were from poor families. During the discussion, the group discussion brought out that the majority of the patients were not in a position to accept their body appearance caused by MDR-TB. Many shared that, due to poor family income, they were not in a position to meet their daily needs. The patients were happy with their relationships with their family members, but their relationships with other family members were poor due to this illness.
- The discussion revealed that the majority of the young people were worried and lost sleep because they had MDR-TB and female participants shared that they were concerned about their future marriage and family life and were worried. The group members were feeling unhappy due to this illness and were not enjoying their day-to-day activities around them. They also shared that this illness had made them lose confidence.
- The group members shared that they were disappointed, embarrassed, and isolated because of their physical appearance and the way they looked, which had kept them away from their friends/neighbours and relatives.
- The MDR-TB patients also shared that they received good care and day-to-day support from family members at the time of illness. Only one patient shared that he did not receive any support from his family members. The participants shared that their family members did not isolate them because of MDR-TB.
- The discussion revealed that most of the participants had taken previous TB treatment in private and had spent money on the treatment and later reached the government health facility. The participants in the group shared that the treatment and diagnosis were free for them from the government health facility. The group discussion also brought out that the patients have received support from government field staff for MDR-TB coordinators.

- Except for two patients, all the others in the group had taken TB treatment earlier. Except for one patient, all of them had gone for private TB treatment and spent money on the treatment afterwards.
- FGD interview participants MDR-TB patients' names were not mentioned anywhere in this book for the confidentiality of the book participants.

4. *Focus Group Discussion—South Chennai*

Venue: Lalithapuram TB unit, Chennai.

No of participants: 08 (5 Men and 3 Women)

The focus group discussion was held at Lalithapuram TB unit, Chennai, between 8.30 and 10 am. Five men and three women participated in the discussion; the participants were in the age group of 20 to 55 years old. The discussion was divided into two sessions of 45 minutes each, with a 15-minute break in-between.

The FGD focused on general health status and well-being, stigma, family support, treatment and available support systems for MDR-TB patients.

The following were the outcomes of the FGD:

- The MDR-TB patients shared that they were not satisfied with their health condition due to TB illness. Except for one patient, all of them lived in a poor housing environment and they were from poor socio-economic status. Most of the patients were not in a position to accept their physical appearance due to MDR-TB. The majority of the patients shared that they did not have sufficient money to meet their daily needs. The respondents shared that the personal relationships in the patient's family were good and the relationships outside the family remained poor due to this illness.
- The FGD also revealed that young people had lost their sleep, especially the female group members. They were the ones who had mostly lost their sleep worrying about MDR-TB. They were feeling unhappy and they were not enjoying their day-to-day activities. They felt that they were losing confidence.

- The discussions also revealed that the majority of the young patients were the ones who were isolated, disappointed, and embarrassed because of their physical appearance due to TB, which distanced them from their friends, neighbours, and relatives.
- The other important information revealed by the participants was that the patients received support from their family members for their day-to-day activities during the illness. They also shared that they were not isolated by their family because of their TB illness.
- It was obvious to note from the discussion that the participants had taken previous TB treatment and they had spent money on private TB treatment before going to government hospitals.
- The discussion revealed that the patients had availed of free TB treatment and diagnostic facilities from the government. The participants were not aware of the NGO's support. One of the participants shared that an NGO coordinator used to come to meet him to see if he was taking treatment properly and providc treatment advice.

Focus Group Discussion—West Chennai

Venue: Thiruvanmiyur TB Unit-Chennai.

No of participants: 9 (6 Men and 3 Women).

The authors conducted the focus group discussion. The FGD was conducted at Thiruvanmiyur TB Unit-Chennai from 10.00 am to 12.00 noon. Nine MDR-TB patients participated in the discussion; among them, 6 were men and 3 were women. The participants were in the age group between 25 and 65 years old. The session was divided into two sessions of 45 minutes each, with a 30-minute break in-between.

The identified questions on the focus areas of general health status and well-being, stigma, patient family support, treatment-related issues and the available support systems for them were discussed.

The discussions brought out the following points;

- Most of the group members shared that they were not satisfied with their current health condition because of MDR-TB. The discussion also brought out that the majority of the patients' living conditions were poor and their family status was poor. Except for two patients, all the patients shared that they were not in a position to accept their bodily appearance caused by MDR-TB.

- The discussions also brought out that Most of the patients' socioeconomic condition was poor and they lived on a shoestring budget, not enough to meet their daily needs. The patients shared that their relationship with their family members was OK and some of them said it was good, but the majority shared that their relationship outside the family was not so good due to their illness.
- The female patients shared that they had lost sleep worrying about their condition due to TB. The young people were most worried and lost their sleep. They felt dejected and did not enjoy their day-to-day activities. They also lost their confidence.
- The discussion also brought out that the majority of the young patients were isolated, disappointed and embarrassed because of their physical appearance, and they shared that they kept a distance from their friends, neighbours and relatives.
- The patients in the group were happy to share about their family members support during this illness. One of the group members shared that he did not have anyone to take care and he did not have a family. The patients in the group also shared that they were not isolated by the family members because of TB.
- During the discussion, the majority of the group members shared that they had received previous TB treatment from private sources. Many of them had spent money on private TB treatment before approaching government hospitals.
- The participants also shared that they received free treatment and diagnostic support for TB from a government hospital. The participants shared that they were not aware of any NGO or association. Some of the participants shared that they had received support from healthy volunteers or ASHA and also from DoT providers for MDR-TB treatment.

- FGD interview participants MDR-TB patients' names were not mentioned anywhere in this book for the confidentiality of the book participants.

Conclusion

The qualitative data was analysed by using thematic analysis broad domains of general health status and well-being, stigma, patient family support, treatment-related issues and the available support systems for them were discussed. Most of the patients opined that their general health was affected by tuberculosis. Around two-thirds of patients still have the stigma of receiving treatment, accessing health services, and family support. Concerning family support, most patients have support from their spouse and other close relatives, but peer groups are not as supportive as family members. About the treatment issues, government and non-governmental organisations have extended the services. The government has introduced many programmes to treat patients at the central and state level through local health facilities.

The awareness level and support system from the non-governmental organisations were not as expected by the community and the TB patients, except for the dot providers' support felt by the patients, but in contrast to that, the governmental initiatives were enormous than the non-governmental organisations.

To reduce the stigma, non-governmental organisations and social work institutions would provide support to patients through counselling and guidance to the stakeholders for better treatment services. To ensure patients get continuous treatment, non-governmental organisations can initiate and support nutritional support for patients.

CHAPTER 15

MDR-TB Research: Future Directions and Conclusion

Introduction

Drawing from the previous chapter 'Analyses and Interpretations', this chapter highlights the major findings of the book, puts forward potential suggestions, indicates future research directions, and concludes the book. The chapter is presented in four portions, namely Major Findings, Suggestions, Future Directions and Conclusion. The major findings are organised into four sections; viz. the profile of the respondents, 'Analyses and Interpretations'. It is followed by future research directions and then the conclusion of the book.

Major Findings of the Research Study

Demographic and Personal Profile

- Among the total respondents, 72.7 per cent of the respondents were male MDR-TB patients and 27.3 per cent were female MDR-TB patients.
- Among the respondents, Male MDR-TB patients were higher compared to female MDR-TB patients.
- The total number of Male MDR-TB patients were 72.7 per cent. Among the Male MDR-TB patients, in North Chennai were (24.6%), East Chennai (19.7%), Central Chennai (13.8%), West Chennai (7.6%) and South Chennai 6.9 per cent.
- The Female respondent constituted around 27.3 per cent, among them respondents from North Chennai (6.2%), East Chennai (6.9%), Central Chennai (6.6%), West Chennai (4.8%) and South Chennai 2.8 per cent of female MDR-TB patients. It is observed that the Male MDR-TB patients were higher (72.7%)

when compared to the female MDR-TB patients (27.3%) in Chennai Corporation Health Districts.

- It was found that, together, one-fourth of MDR-TB patients in the age groups between 18 and 30 (24.6 per cent) and 51 to 60 (25.3 per cent) were older than the total number of MDR-TB patients in all three districts, which was greater than the total number of MDR-TB patients in all three districts.
- When it is compared among the five districts in Chennai with the age group of the MDR-TB patients, it is found that the majority (30.8%) of the MDR-TB patients were from North Chennai when compared to other districts. Next to North Chennai in the East Chennai were (26.6%) and Central Chennai is had (20.4%) in all the age group.
- It is observed that a lower number of MDR-TB cases were in West Chennai (12.5%) and South Chennai and had below 10 per cent which is lower in all the age groups when compared to the other 3 districts in Chennai.
- The majority of MDR-TB patients (91.7%) in Chennai Corporation's five Health Districts were Hindus. When compared to other religions, Hindus were greater (29.8 per cent) in North Chennai and East Chennai (24.5 per cent). However, the number of MDR-TB patients was lower in Central Chennai (17.6%), West Chennai (11.4%), and South Chennai (8.5%).
- The proportion of patients who belonged to the Muslim community was 5.5%. According to the data. It has been observed that there are no Muslim patients in North Chennai, which is unusual. East and Central Chennai each had 2.1 per cent of the MDR patients, and West and South Chennai each had 0.7 per cent of the MDR patients belonging to the Muslim religion.
- The MDR-TB patients from the Christian community were 2.8 per cent, among them one per cent from North Chennai and 0.7 from Central Chennai. It is observed that East, west and south Chennai are negligible numbers (0.3%) belong to the Christian religion.
- MDR-TB patients are found to be predominantly concentrated in the nuclear family structure (83.0 per cent), according to the

data gathered. Among those, 11.4 per cent were members of a joint family structure, and the remaining 5.5 per cent were not applicable in either category or were inconsequential in either category. One-fourth of those who answered the survey questions (25.3 per cent) are from North Chennai, while 23.2 per cent are from East Chennai.

- A total of 50.9 per cent of those who had three to five members in their family had two members, followed by 6.2 per cent and 4.5 per cent who had more than five members. The proportion of patients who had three to five family members was higher (50.9 per cent) as compared to the other numbers of family members in the MDR-TB patients' households, as can be seen in the chart below:

Socioeconomic Profile

- When asked about their job situation, the MDR-TB patients revealed that the majority (44.3 per cent) of those who answered the book were employed and the remaining (38.1 per cent) were unemployed. Students accounted for 10.4% and 7.3% of them were housewives during their illness.
- Among the respondents 44.3 per cent was employed during their illness and of them from North Chennai16.3 per cent, East Chennai ten per cent, Central Chennai (9.3%), West Chennai (4.5%) per cent and South Chennai were (4.2%) respectively.
- The patients who were unemployed during their illness were 38.1 per cent, among them from North Chennai (10.7) per cent, East Chennai (11.8%), Central Chennai (6.2%), West Chennai (4.8%) per cent and South Chennai were (4.5%) respectively.
- There were no job opportunities available to more than half of those who responded (55.7 per cent). East Chennai had the highest percentage (16.6) in this category, followed by North Chennai (14.5 per cent), Central Chennai (11.1 per cent), West Chennai (eight per cent), and 5.5 per cent from South Chennai, which had the lowest percentage (5.5 per cent). The fact that MDR-TB patients who are not eligible for any employment are virtually always unemployed can be observed, which indicates

that if the breadwinner becomes ill, the family would suffer as a result of a reduction in income.

- When it comes to monthly income or wage, more than half of the patients (56.1 per cent) reported that they received none during their sickness. Their home district was East Chennai, which accounted for 16.6 per cent of them, followed by North Chennai (14.5 per cent), and Central Chennai (14 per cent) (11.4 per cent). Low-income neighbourhoods in West Chennai (8.0 per cent) and South Chennai (8.0 per cent) are particularly prevalent (5.5 per cent).
- It can be seen that more than half (55.7 per cent) of them make more than Rs. 10000, and a quarter (27 per cent) earn between Rs. 5001 and Rs. 10000. It has also been shown that one-fifth of people who have studied up to higher education earn Rs. 10000/- or more.
- It can be observed that 17.3 per cent of the patient's family income was less than Rs. 5000/-per month, which indicates a financial hardship. It was twenty-seven per cent of the patient's family's monthly income, which ranged from Rs. 5001 to Rs. 10,000/-. An estimated 55.7 per cent of the patient's household earned more than Rs. 10000/- each year.
- Approximately two-thirds (63.3 per cent) of the respondents had a single earning member in their family, with 19.7 per cent living in North Chennai, 17.3 per cent living in East Chennai, 13.1 per cent living in Central Chennai, 6.9 per cent living in West Chennai, and 5.9 per cent living in South Chennai.
- It should be noted that the proportion of MDR-TB patients from single-member earning families was high, implying that if the breadwinner becomes ill, the family will suffer from the loss of income that results. Second, there will be additional expenses for MDR-TB patients, which will have to be covered by the income of the sole member of the family.
- The vast majority (38.4 per cent) of patients lived in their own houses. The percentage of patients who lived in rented housing was 28.7%. Patients who held a lease on a home were (13.5 per cent). Patients who did not have access to a home or who stated

that the housing style they preferred was not appropriate were grouped (19.4).

- It has been found that more than half (51.9 per cent) of MDR-TB patients have paid monthly house rent, with 11.8 per cent endorsing from North Chennai, 13.5 per cent hailing from East Chennai, 13.1 per cent hailing from Central Chennai, 8.7 per cent hailing from West Chennai, and 4.8% hailing from South Chennai.

TB and MDR-TB Treatment Profile

- 40.5 per cent of tuberculosis patients said that they were sick for less than a year.
- More than half of these were patients who had been unwell for one to two years (59.5 per cent).
- The age and duration of MDR-TB therapy were seen to be between 1 and 2 years, with seventeen per cent belonging to the age group of 18 to 30 years, followed by 14.9 per cent belonging to the age group of 51 to 60 years.
- 21.1 Per cent of respondents with MDR tuberculosis had spent money on the diagnosis of tuberculosis and another condition.
- 14.9% had spent money on meals to treat tuberculosis and other sickness.
- 17% had spent money on food items while undergoing MDR-TB therapy.
- The vast majority (47.1%) of patients spent money on travel expenses while undergoing MDR-TB treatment.
- It shows that those who have struggled with MDR-TB treatment can benefit from it. According to the total responders, 14.5 per cent of MDR-TB patients experienced harmful side effects. They had financial challenges in 28 per cent of cases. Social problems affect 9.3% of patients. During MDR-TB therapy, 48.1 per cent of respondents (the majority) said they had no problems.
- It is observed that there is a correlation between MDR-TB patients' feelings throughout therapy and those who have better sensations during treatment (41.5 per cent). Among them, the

majority (16.6) came from North Chennai, while 9.7 per cent came from East Chennai. East Chennai (11.4 per cent) and central Chennai (10 per cent) share the same sentiment.

Family Support Profile

- It can be seen that the majority of MDR-TB patients (75.4%) did not receive support from their families during their TB disease.
- The majority of the respondents (61.6%) stated that they were isolated by their family members as a result of their MDR-TB. Some respondents (38.4%) claimed that they were not isolated from their family members.
- Most of the respondents (61.6 per cent) reported that they were sleeping separately from their family members due to MDR-TB.
- MDR-TB patients were sleeping with their family members during their MDR-TB disease, according to some (38.4) responders.
- It's been reported that 46.7 per cent of MDR-TB patients have daily meals with their families, while 53.31 per cent of respondents said they were given food separately owing to their TB sickness.
- The majority of responders (58.8%) did not separate the glass and plate when eating meals with their families.
- Due to their TB disease, 41.2 per cent of MDR-TB patients were observed abusing broken glass and plates to take their food home provided by their family members.
- Twenty-six per cent of the patients were from North Chennai, 14.2 per cent from East Chennai, 16.3 per cent from West Chennai, 10.4 per cent from East Chennai, and 8.7% from South Chennai.

Institutional Support

- It was reported that more than half (53.3%) of the MDR-TB patients reported that the nearest government health facility was more than 5 kilometres away from their residence. Of the total number of responders, 46.7% stated that the nearest government health facility or government hospital is less than 5 kilometres away.

- A total of 51.9 per cent of patients felt that the service provided by the government-run healthcare facility was satisfactory. 15 per cent came from North Chennai, 12 per cent from East Chennai, 11 per cent from Central Chennai, 7 per cent from West Chennai, and 4.5 per cent came from South Chennai. The respondents did not mention that they were unable to express any thoughts regarding the government health facility and its services.

Health Facility

- It was revealed that more than half (58.1%) of the MDR-TB patients reported that the behaviour of government health workers and the quality of their treatment at the government health facility were satisfactory. Patients who were satisfied with the behaviour of government health workers and the quality of their treatment accounted for 41.9% of the total.
- The distribution of health services in the Greater Chennai Corporation (GCC) is shown by the health district. The majority (30.8%) of the MDR-TB patients were from North Chennai, with 26.6 per cent coming from East Chennai, according to the data. Central Chennai contributed 20.4 per cent, West Chennai contributed 12.5 per cent, and South Chennai contributed 9.7 per cent. A majority (6.6%) of the MDR-TB patients were from Kodungaiyur and the East Coast Road (ECR) TB units. Thiruvottriur 5.5 per cent, Pulianthope 4.5 per cent.
- It was reported that more than half (53.3%) of the MDR-TB patients stated that the nearest government health facility was more than 5 kilometres away from their residence.
- In all, 46.7% of those who answered the survey stated that the nearest government health institution or government hospital is fewer than 5 kilometres away.
- 9 per cent were the majority of patients who shared the satisfaction of the public health facility service. Of those, 15.9% were from North Chennai, 12.8% were from East Chennai, 11.1% were from Central Chennai, 11.6% were from West

Chennai, and 4.5% were from South Chennai. The respondents did not say that their views about government health facilities and their services could not be expressed.

- Most patients who shared the satisfactoriness of the government health institution were 51.9%. Of those, 15.9% were from North Chennai, 12.8% were from East Chennai, 11.1% were from Central Chennai, 11.6% were from West Chennai, and 4.5% were from South Chennai. The respondents did not express their views about the government health institution and its services.
- Over half (58.1) of MDR-TB patients reported that the behaviour and service of government health personnel in government healthcare institutions were good. Patients who discussed satisfactory behaviour and service with government health workers were 41.9%.

Psychological Well-being (PWB) of MDR-TB Patients

Level of Autonomy

- The majority of patients in government health institution satisfactory conditions were 51.9 per cent. Of these, 15.9% were from Chennai North, 12.8% were from Chennai East, 11.1% were from Chennai central, 11,6% were from Chennai West, and 4.5% were from South Chennai South. The interviewees did not voice their views about the state health institution and its services.
- More than half (58.1) MDR-TB patients reported that the behaviour and service of government staff were good in public health. 41,9% of patients had positive behaviour and good service in their discussions with health care personnel.
- Among the female respondents, 27.3% of respondents showed a low level of autonomy, and 5.5% of those individuals exhibited a moderate level of autonomy. However, evidence of a moderate level of autonomy was observed in 18.0% of patients and 3.8% of patients.
- As patients aged 41 to 50, the proportion of people with a low degree of autonomy was 22.5 per cent of the total, those with a

Moderate level of autonomy were 15.2 per cent, and those with a high level of autonomy were 4.5 per cent.

- Patients aged 51 to 60 years old constituted 25.3 per cent of the total, with 8% having a low level of autonomy, 14.9 per cent having a moderate level of autonomy, and 2.4 per cent having a high level of autonomy. Patients over the age of 60 accounted for 13.1 per cent of the total, with 4.5 per cent having a low level of autonomy, 7.6 per cent having a moderate level of autonomy, and one per cent having a high level of autonomy. When compared to other age groups, MDR-TB patients in this age range were the most afflicted.
- Of the 91.7 per cent of patients who identified as Hindu, 24.2 per cent had a low level of autonomy; however, evidence of a moderate level of autonomy was found in 54.3 per cent, and 13.1 per cent had a high level of autonomy. Patients who practised Islam made up 5.5 per cent of the total, with one per cent having a low and high level of autonomy and 3.5 per cent having a moderate level of autonomy. Christian patients made up 2.8 per cent of the total, with (0.3) per cent having a low level of autonomy, 2.4 per cent having a moderate level of autonomy, and none having a high level of autonomy.
- Those who had studied up to primary school, high school, and higher secondary demonstrated indications of a moderate level of autonomy in psychological well-being (10.7 per cent), (19.7%), and (12.5 per cent) accordingly.
- Among the 69.2 per cent of patients who had married, 15.6 per cent had a low level of autonomy, 43.9 per cent had a moderate level of autonomy, and 9.7% had a high level of autonomy. The majority of the respondents were married, and nearly half of those who were married showed signs of moderate autonomy.
- It is observed that half of MDR-TB patients were (50.9%) living with 3 to 5 family members among them there is evidence of a moderate level of autonomy (32.2%) in the psychological well-being of MDR-TB patients.
- It was found that more than half of MDR-TB patients (63.0 per cent) lived with only one earning family member, indicating a

modest level of autonomy (38.1 per cent) in the psychological well-being of MDR-TB patients.

- It can be seen that those MDR-TB patients who were employed (44.3%) had a moderate level of autonomy, while those who were unemployed (29.8%) had a low level of autonomy (38.1 per cent). According to their employment situation, 21.1 per cent of them have a moderate level of psychological autonomy.
- The association between the monthly income and the degree of self-sufficiency of MDR-tub patients (56.1%) were due to MDR-TB and unable to get to work (30.8%) had to be noticed as a result that their income level was modestly autonomous. It reveals that people with MDR-TB have been unable to routinely work with therapy due to long-term significant adverse effects.
- In the table above, it is seen that almost one fifth (24.2 per cent) of patients with a greater sense of illness due to MDR-TB indicated a moderate level of autonomy depending on their feelings about illness, due to MDR (41.5%) and the autonomy level of MDR-TB patients. One fifth (22.1%) per cent of the patients who had the same feelings about the illness (37.7 per cent) had moderate autonomy according to their sense of illness.
- The type of difficulty and the amount of autonomy of patients with MDR-TB can be observed from the table above. Those with economic difficulties were 28%, of which eighteen% showed a moderate level of autonomy. There was (48.1 per cent) evidence of a moderate level of autonomy in patients with additional issues of 29.1 per cent.
- The relationship between the support of families and the level of independence of patients with MDR-TB is observed.
- 2 per cent of the patients who received support from a family member were (24.6) MDR, with moderate autonomy evidence.
- Patients who did not get help from a family member were (75.4) 45 per cent of them, according to the support of their family member, had moderate autonomy proof.

Level of Environmental Mastery

- 72.7 per cent (10.4) of those who were male had a low environmental mastery level. However, there was a moderate self-acceptance level (46.7) per cent of the patients and a high level of environmental mastery for 10.4 per cent of the patients. The female responders represented 27.3%. 5.5 per cent of them have a low degree of environmental skills. There was, however, a moderate level of self-acceptance among (18.3) patients and a high level of environmental mastership among (3.5 per cent of patients).

- The patients' ages ranged from 18 to 30 years (24.6) and 31 to 40 years (34.6). (22.5). 16.3 per cent of people in both age groups showed a moderate level of self-acceptance.
- Religion and MDR-TB patients' level of self-acceptance according to religion The Hindu patients made up 91.7 per cent of the total. One-fourth (14.5%) of them exhibited a low level of environmental mastery. However, evidence of a moderate level of self-acceptance was found in 58.8 per cent (18.3%) of those with a high level of environmental mastery.
- It was reported that those who had completed elementary, high school, and higher secondary school had evidence of a moderate level of self-acceptance in psychological well-being (14.5%), (20.1%), and 13.1%, respectively.
- Of the 69.2% of patients who married, 19.7% had a low level of Environmental Mastery, 45.7 per cent had a moderate level of self-acceptance, and 13.8% had a high level of Environmental Mastery.
- The majority of respondents (69.2 per cent) were married, and nearly half (45.7 per cent) of those who were married demonstrated signs of a moderate level of environ
- Most (83%) of them lived in nuclear families, it is observed.
- Half of them showed a moderate level of environmental mastery.
- Of the above data, it was noticed that half (50.9%) of patients with MDR-TB lived with between 3 and 5 family members.
- The psychological health of MDR-TB patients showed moderate levels of self-acceptance (30,8%).
- Half of MDR-TBe patients (44.3%) and unemployed (27.7%) reported a moderate level of self-acceptance in their psychological

well-being based on their employment status.50.9% of MDR-TB patients (50.9%) have three to five family members.

- More than half of MDR-TB patients (50.9 per cent) live with three to five family members.
- As indicated in the preceding table, patients who worked in other sectors (55.7 per cent) and those who worked in other sectors (37.4 per cent) demonstrated a moderate level of self-acceptance in terms of psychological well-being,
- The accompanying table demonstrates a relationship between the style of dwelling in which MDR-TB patients live and their level of self-acceptance. Those who lived in their own home (38.4 per cent) compared to those who were suffering from MDR (23.9 per cent) had a moderate level of self-acceptance, depending on the type of home.
- The association between patients' perceptions of the condition and their amount of autonomy is seen in the preceding table. Among those who reported having more positive feelings regarding the disease (41.5%), nearly a fifth (24.2%) had a moderate level of autonomy concerning their disease-related feelings. Among patients who had a similar perception of the disease (37.7 per cent) due to MDR, one-fifth (22.1 per cent) demonstrated a moderate level of autonomy about their perception of the disease.
- It is noted that MDR-TB patients have a variety of problems and a low level of self-acceptance.
- Twenty-eight per cent of respondents reported having an economic problem.
- 15.9 per cent of them had a moderate level of self-acceptance.
- Patients with co-occurring disorders were (48.1 per cent).
- 31.8 per cent of them demonstrated a moderate level of environmental competence
- It is noted that the majority of respondents, 75.4 per cent, report having no family support.
- 48.1 per cent of patients had a Moderate Level of Environmental Mastery.

Level of Personal Growth

- Most of the respondents (72.7% of them) were male.
- Forty-six per cent of respondents indicated that there was moderate personal growth.
- Among the patients between the ages of 18 and 30, 24.6% demonstrated a moderate level of personal progress.
- Among those who were aged from 51 to 60, those with a moderate level of personal progress represented (25.3%) of those with this age range.
- Christian had 2.8% of the patients.
- About 1.7% of people in the book fell into the category of those with a low level of personal growth, about 17.4% fell into the category of those with a moderate level of personal growth, and only 1.4% of people had a high level of personal growth.
- The figures show that of those who have completed high school, 33.2% obtained a post-secondary education.
- Close to one fifth (19.0%) of these people (i.e., nearly one-fifth of the group) exhibit indications of moderate personal progress.
- Only 23.9 per cent revealed evidence of moderate personal growth, and of this group, only half (20.4 per cent) revealed evidence of moderate personal progress (20.8 per cent).
- About 14.2% of those who took the assessment had achieved a moderate level of personal progress.
- It has been found that people infected with MDR-TB form families and demonstrate greater personal growth than those not infected.
- Approximately 83% of these people are living in nuclear families.
- Including roughly half of them, around half of the group had shown evidence of having experienced a moderate level of personal growth.
- Half of MDR-TB patients (50.9 per cent) live with three to five family members.
- Among them, there is evidence of a moderate level of personal growth (30.4%) in MDR-TB patients' psychological well-being.

- According to the above table, MDR-TB patients who have employed 44.3 per cent, 25.6 per cent of whom had evidence of a moderate level of personal progress.
- As a result, the unemployed (38.1%) had evidence of a modest level of personal progress, whereas the employed (25.6%) did not.
- As a result, both employed and employed people had identical levels of personal improvement
- According to the above data, MDR patients working in other sectors accounted for more than half (55.7%) of them, and one-third (36.0%) of them had evidence of a moderate level of personal progress in psychological well-being based on their employment sector.
- The relationship between monthly income and the amount of personal growth of MDR-TB patients can be seen in the table above, with more than half of them (56.1%) having no income. According to their income level, 30.8 per cent of them showed indications of a moderate level of personal growth. It demonstrates that MDR-TB patients were unable to work regularly due to the treatment's long duration and adverse effects.
- The association between MDR-TB patients' attitudes about the disease and their level of personal progress may be seen in the above table. There were fewer than half of those who had positive feelings towards the condition (41.5 per cent). According to their better feelings regarding the sickness, 24.9 per cent of those who had better feelings had evidence of a moderate level of personal progress. Patients who felt the same way about their illness were grouped (37.7 per cent). According to their identical feelings about the sickness, over a quarter (23.9%) of them had evidence of a moderate level of personal growth.
- The types of issues and personal growth of MDR-TB patients can be shown in the table above. Twenty-eight per cent of those polled said they were having financial difficulties. Eighteen per cent of them showed signs of moderate personal development. Patients with a variety of issues were included in the book (48.1 per cent). Among them, 29.1% showed signs of moderate personal development.

Level of a Positive Relationship

- The majority (72.7 per cent) of respondents were male, and there was evidence of a moderate level of a good relationship, with almost half (46.4 per cent) of respondents having a favourable relationship.
- Patients aged 18 to 30 years had a 24.6 per cent positive relationship, with 15.9 per cent having a moderate degree of a positive relationship, while those aged 51 to 60 years had a 25.3 per cent positive relationship, with 16.6 per cent having a moderate degree of a positive relationship.
- Although the majority of patients (91.7%) were Hindu, evidence of a moderate level of favourable associations was observed in more than half of them (55.7%).
- It is noticed that 33.2 per cent of individuals who have completed high school (18.7 per cent) exhibit evidence of a moderate level of a positive association.
- 69.2 per cent of patients were married, and the majority (39.1 per cent) of this group had a moderate level of positive relationships, whereas the unmarried patients were (20.8 per cent). 13.8 per cent of them reported having a moderate level of favourable relationships.
- The vast majority, 83%, lived in nuclear families. Almost half (47.8 per cent) of them demonstrated a moderate level of a positive association. In comparison to the combined family, there was only 8% evidence of a moderate level of a positive relationship. This demonstrates that the combined family benefited from family assistance to maintain a strong relationship.
- More than half of MDR-TB patients (50.9 per cent) lived with three to five family members. Among them, there is evidence of a moderately good link with 31.5 per cent of MDR-TB patients' psychological well-being.
- It is shown in the preceding table that MDR-TB patients who were employed (44.3%) and those who were jobless (28.7 per cent) had a modest level of a positive association, but MDR-TB patients who were unemployed (38.1). Almost one-fifth (21.8

per cent) of them shown a moderate level of positive link with psychological well-being concerning their employment situation.

- More than half (55.7 per cent) of MDR patients worked in other sectors, and one-third (30.4) of them demonstrated a moderate level of favourable link with psychological well-being based on their employment sector.
- More than half of MDR-TB patients (56.1%) did not have a source of income, whereas 30.4 per cent demonstrated a moderately good relationship with their income level. MDR-TB patients were unable to work regularly due to the prolonged duration and unanticipated outcomes.
- The relationship between disease sensitivity and positive relationships in MDR-TB patients revealed that those who felt better about the disease were less than half (41.5%), with approximately one-fourth feeling better and (24.9%) having evidence of a moderate level of positive relationships consistent with their improved feelings about the disease.
- 48.1 per cent of patients experienced additional difficulties during treatment for MDR-TB, including 14.9 per cent who had a low level of positive relationships, 28.7 per cent who had a moderate level of positive relationships, and 4.5 who had a high degree of positive relationships.
- One-fourth of patients (24.6 per cent) received assistance from family members, and 14.9 per cent demonstrated a moderately positive relationship. Seventy-five per cent (75.4 per cent) of patients reported receiving no assistance from family members, whereas 44.3% reported having moderately pleasant interactions.

Level of the Purpose of Life

- The majority of respondents, 72.7 per cent, were male, and there was evidence of a moderate level of purpose in life, with almost half (45.7%) of respondents indicating a moderate level of life purpose. When compared to females, there is evidence of a moderate level of purpose in life among 27.3 per cent of them and 14.5 per cent.

- It is observed that the patients who were aged between 18 to 30 years were (24.6%) and among them (14.5%) had a moderate level of purpose in life, and the patients who were aged between 51 to 60 years were (25.3%) and among them (13.8%) had a moderate level of purpose in life.
- It is observed that those who have studied up to high school are 33.2 per cent. Among them, nearly one fifth (19.0%) have evidence of a moderate level of purpose in life.
- The patients who were married were 69.2 per cent and among this group, the majority (39.1%) of them had a moderate level of purpose in life, whereas the unmarried patients were (20.8%). Among them, 13.8 per cent had a moderate level of purpose in life.
- The majority, 83% of them, living in a nuclear family. Among them, nearly half (49.5%) had evidence of a moderate level of the purpose of life. When compared to the joint family, which had only 7.3 per cent. This shows that the joint family had family support in connection with the level of the purpose of life.
- It is observed that half of the MDR-TB patients (50.9%) were living with 3 to 5 family members. Among them, there is evidence of a moderate level of the purpose of life of 31.8 per cent of MDR-TB patients.
- It is observed that MDR-TB patients who were employed were (44.3) and among them (25.3%) had evidence of a moderate level of purpose in life, whereas MDR-TB patients who were unemployed were (38.1). Among them, nearly one fifth (23.5%) had evidence of a moderate level of purpose in life.
- It is observed that MDR-TB patients who were working as labour/daily wages were (25.3) and among them (14.9) had evidence of a moderate level of purpose in life, whereas MDR-TB patients who were not working any place/company were (55.7%). Among them, nearly one-fifth of them (34.9%) had evidence of a moderate level of purpose in life.
- According to the preceding statistics, more than half of the MDR-TB patients (56.1%) had no income, whereas 35.3 per cent revealed evidence of a moderate level of purpose in life with

their income level. Due to the longer duration and unexpected consequences, MDR-TB patients were unable to work regularly.

- It is observed the kinds of problems and personal growth of MDR-TB patients. Those who had economic problems were twenty-eight per cent. Among them, 29.1 per cent had evidence of moderate personal growth. Patients who have other problems were (48.1%). Among them, 29.1 per cent had evidence of moderate personal growth.
- One-fourth of the patients (24.6%) had family member support, and 14.9 per cent showed evidence of a somewhat positive relationship. Three-quarters (75.4%) of the patients reported no assistance from family members, whereas 48.8 per cent had a moderate level of purpose in the life of MDR-TB patients.

Level of Self-Acceptance

- When compared to females, there is evidence of a Moderate level of psychological well-being among them (18.7).
- It is noticed that patients aged 18 to 30 years had a moderate level of self-acceptance (24.6%) and patients aged 51 to 60 years had a moderate level of self-acceptance (25.3%) and 13.8% had a moderate level of self-acceptance.
- The majority of respondents (72.7 per cent) were male, and almost half (40.1 per cent) of respondents reported having a moderate level of self-acceptance.
- It is noted that 33.2 per cent of them studied up to the high school level. Nearly a fifth (20.1%) of them had evidence of a high level of self-acceptance, compared to 10% of those who had studied up to undergrad, with 6.2 per cent of them having evidence of a high level of self-acceptance.
- 2 per cent of patients were married, and the majority (40.1 per cent) of these patients demonstrated a moderate level of self-acceptance, whereas unmarried patients demonstrated a low level of self-acceptance (20.8 per cent).
- 12.5 per cent of them reported having a moderate level of self-acceptance.

- The majority of MDR-TB patients (83%) live in nuclear families, with half (50.9%) having evidence of a moderate level of self-acceptance. In comparison, the joint family population was 11.4 per cent, with only 5.2 per cent having evidence of a moderate level of self-acceptance.
- As seen in the preceding table, more than half (50.9 per cent) of MDR tuberculosis patients lived with three to five family members. Among them, there is evidence of a moderate level of self-acceptance (31.5%) among MDR-TB patients' psychological well-being.
- MDR-TB patients who were employed (44.3 per cent) had a moderate degree of self-acceptance, whereas MDR-TB patients who were jobless (38.1 per cent) had a moderate level of self-acceptance (22.8 per cent).
- MDR-TB patients who worked as labour/daily wage were (25.3 per cent), and 13.5 per cent of them had evidence of a moderate level of the purpose of life, whereas MDR-TB patients who did not work were (55.7 per cent), and more than one-third (33.6 per cent) of them had evidence of a moderate level of the purpose of life.
- MDR-TB patients who worked as labour/daily wage were (25.3 per cent), and 13.5 per cent of them had evidence of a moderate level of the purpose of life, whereas MDR-TB patients who did not work were (55.7 per cent), and more than one-third (33.6 per cent) of them had evidence of a moderate level of the purpose of life.
- More than half of MDR-TB patients (56.1%) did not have a source of income, whereas 33.9 per cent demonstrated a moderately good relationship with their income level.
- MDR-TB patients were unable to work regularly due to the prolonged duration and unanticipated outcomes.
- 48.1 per cent of patients experienced additional difficulties during treatment for MDR-TB, including 5.9 per cent who had a low degree of self-acceptance, 29.8 per cent who had a moderate level of self-acceptance, and 12.5 per cent who had a high level of self-acceptance.

- One-fourth of patients (24.6 per cent) received assistance from family members, and 15.9 per cent demonstrated a moderately positive relationship. 75.4 per cent of patients reported receiving no aid from family members, whereas 42.9 per cent reported having a moderate level of self-acceptance.

Level of Psychological Well-being

- The majority of respondents (72.7 per cent) were male, and there was evidence of a moderate level of psychological well-being, with almost half (40.5 per cent) reporting a sense of well-being. When compared to females, 27.3 per cent of them exhibit signs of moderate psychological well-being (17.3 per cent).
- It is noted that patients aged 18 to 30 years were (24.6%) and (15.2% of them had a moderate level of psychological well-being, while those aged 51 to 60 years were (25.3%) and (15.2% of them had a moderate level of psychological well-being.
- It is noted that 33.2 per cent of them studied up to the high school level. Nearly one-fifth (17.6%) of them demonstrated a moderate level of psychological well-being.
- 69.2 per cent, of whom 39.8 per cent had moderate psychological well-being, whereas those who were not married were 78.4 per cent (20.8 per cent). Approximately 12.1% of the group (some 785 individuals) reported moderate psychological well-being.
- Over eighty-three per cent of the people lived in nuclear families. Moreover, half (47.4%) of the group had moderate indications of psychological well-being. an 11.4% difference as compared to the united family. However, of those who tested positive, only 8% showed indications of a modest level of psychological well-being. Family support in connection with a positive relationship is implied by this finding.
- Approximately half of the MDR-TB patients (50.9 per cent) had at least 3-5 family members living with them. This book also shows that the psychological well-being of MDR-TB patients is on the lower end, with a score of 30.4%.

- Employed patients (44.3 per cent) and unemployed patients (26.6 per cent) showed signs of a moderate level of psychological well-being according to the statistics above.
- Patients who worked as daily wage or labour were 25.3% and 11.4% respectively and, although that was the case, those who didn't have jobs were 55.7% and nearly one-third (31.8%) were diagnosed with psychological well-being that met the criteria for moderate.
- Data shows that the majority of MDR-TB patients (56.1%) were impoverished, while 32.2% were financially comfortable and emotionally well-off. Income level appears to have a relatively favourable association with the amount of influence it has on their personal lives. Patients infected with MDR-TB found themselves unable to work regularly due to the prolonged duration and unknown outcomes.
- About the condition, one-fourth of the patients agreed (37.7 per cent). (22.8%.) Approximately 60% of people believe they have the same symptoms as the person with the illness, which demonstrates that they have a moderate level of psychological well-being.
- Using the following table, you can determine the problem kind and level of psychological well-being. become resistant to prescribed anti-tuberculosis drugs (MDR-TB). Fifteen.9 per cent of those polled had a moderate level of psychological anguish, while 26.4 per cent had troubles with money. Approximately 48.1% of patients in the book had additional difficulties, and over 30.1% had moderate psychological discomfort.
- 15.6% of patients experienced mild mental well-being, while 24.6% received assistance from family members. 74.4% of patients reported no family member assistance, while 42.2% reported having a moderate level of psychological well-being.

General Health Status of MDR-TB Patients

- Male respondents accounted for 72.7 per cent of the total. 26.6 per cent of them experienced severe prejudice, while 34.3 per cent experienced moderate discrimination. The remaining 11.8 per cent of male patients experienced minimal discrimination.

Female responders made up 27.3% of the total. 13.5 per cent of them had a high level, 10.4 per cent had a moderate level, and 3.5 per cent had a low level.

- 91.7 per cent of Hindus had multidrug-resistant tuberculosis. Seven per cent of patients had a high level of discrimination, 40.8 per cent of Hindus had a moderate level of discrimination, and the remaining 13.8 per cent of Hindus had a low level of discrimination. Muslims accounted for 5.5 per cent of MDR-TB patients. 3.4 per cent of them had a high level of. 6.2 per cent of respondents reported having a moderate level of. 9.1% of them reported having a low level of alienation. Christians made for 2.8 per cent of MDR-TB cases. 1.7 per cent had a high level of estrangement, whereas 1% had a moderate level of alienation. There was no indication of a low level of estrangement.
- 33.2 per cent of patients met the requirements for high school (Metric). 14.2 per cent of them experienced a high sense of alienation. The majority (15.2) of them experienced moderate levels of self-alienation, while the remaining 3.8 per cent experienced minimal levels of alienation. Patients who had completed secondary education (12th class) accounted for 19.7% of the total. 7.3 per cent of these patients had a high level of estrangement, 9% had a moderate level of alienation, and 3.5% had a low level of alienation.
- 4.5 per cent of patients had more than five family members. 2.4 per cent of them reported a high level of estrangement, 1.7% reported a moderate level of alienation, and 0.3% reported a low level of alienation.
- Twenty-eight per cent of respondents were unmarried. 6.6 per cent of them had a high level of estrangement, 11.8 per cent demonstrated a moderate level of alienation, and 2.4 per cent demonstrated a low level of alienation. 69.2 per cent of patients were married, and 30.1 per cent had a high level of estrangement, 28.0% had a moderate level of alienation, and 11.1 per cent had a low level of alienation.
- Moreover half (55.7 per cent) of respondents were unemployed. In this group, 22.5% of patients had a high level of alienation,

25.3% had a moderate level of self-stigma, and 8.0%) had a low level of alienation.

- When this relationship was examined, it was found that the vast majority of respondents (61.6 per cent) reported feeling estranged from their family members as a result of MDR-TB. 23% of participants reported severe alienation as a result of their MDR-TB condition, while 11.4 per cent reported having a very low level of alienation.

Internalized Stigma of Mental Illness

Level of Alienation

- Male respondents accounted for 72.7 per cent of the total. 26.6 per cent of them experienced severe prejudice, while 34.3 per cent experienced moderate discrimination. The remaining 11.8 per cent of male patients experienced minimal discrimination. Female responders made up 27.3% of the total. 13.5 per cent of them had a high level, 10.4 per cent had a moderate level, and 3.5 per cent had a low level.
- 7 per cent of Hindus had multidrug-resistant tuberculosis. Seven per cent of patients had a high level of discrimination, 40.8 per cent of Hindus had a moderate level of discrimination, and the remaining 13.8 per cent of Hindus had a low level of discrimination.
- Muslims accounted for 5.5 per cent of MDR-TB patients. 3.4 per cent of them had a high level of alienation. A moderate level was reported by 6.2 per cent of respondents. 9.1% of them reported having a low level of alienation.
- Christians made for 2.8 per cent of MDR-TB cases. 1.7 per cent had a high level of estrangement, whereas 1% had a moderate level of alienation. There was no indication of a low level of estrangement.
- 2 per cent of patients met the requirements for high school (Metric). 14.2 per cent of them experienced a high sense of alienation. The majority (15.2) of them experienced moderate levels of self-alienation, while the remaining 3.8 per cent

experienced minimal levels of alienation. Patients who had completed secondary education (12th class) accounted for 19.7% of the total. 7.3 per cent of these patients had a high level of estrangement, 9% had a moderate level of alienation, and 3.5% had a low level of alienation.

- Five per cent of patients had more than five family members. 2.4 per cent of them reported a high level of estrangement, 1.7% reported a moderate level of alienation, and 0.3 reported a low level of alienation.
- Twenty-eight per cent of respondents were unmarried. There was a high level of estrangement in 6.6 per cent of them, a moderate level of alienation in 11.8 per cent, and a low level of alienation in 2.4 per cent.69.2 per cent of patients were married, and 30.1 per cent had a high level of estrangement, 28.0% had a moderate level of alienation, and 11.1 per cent had a low level of alienation.
- As seen in the preceding table, more than half (55.7 per cent) of the respondents were unemployed. In this group, 22.5% of patients had a high level of alienation, 25.3% had a moderate level of self-stigma, and 8.0%) had a low level of alienation.
- When this relationship was examined, it was found that the vast majority of respondents (61.6 per cent) reported feeling estranged from their family members as a result of MDR-TB. 23% of participants reported severe alienation as a result of their MDR-TB condition, while 11.4 per cent reported having a very low level of alienation.

Level of Stereotype

A correlation was found between respondents' marital status and their attitudes toward MDR tuberculosis. In the sample, 69.2 per cent were married, with a substantial proportion (30.5 per cent) having stereotypes, while others had moderate (24.9 per cent) or low (16.7 per cent) stereotypes.

- It was observed that individuals with MDR-TB who were employed faced a risk of developing moderate prejudices (44.3).

27,7% of the unemployed demonstrated a moderate level of stereotypes.

- The preceding table demonstrates unequivocally that more than half (55.7 per cent) of respondents were unable to acquire employment. 383 of them had a low level of stereotype, 273 had a moderate level, and 9.7 had a high level.

One-fifth of people (21.5%) revealed evidence of exposure to stereotypes, while another fourth (24.2%) demonstrated symptoms consistent with moderate stereotyping.

Level of Discrimination

- The age and level of discrimination were observed among respondents. Out of the age group of 18 to 30, the patients with MDR tuberculosis were 24.6% with 8.3% having low discrimination, and 3.8% and 12.5% had a moderate level of discrimination.
- Nearly nine out of 10 respondents (89.7%) identified as Hindu, whereas about forty per cent (41.9%) of the Hindus who took part in the survey said they had experienced more discrimination than Muslims and Christians. Muslims were estimated to constitute approximately 5.5% of the population. The reported discrimination incidents differed somewhat between groups: roughly 3.1% of those reporting had high levels of discrimination, while the remaining 2.8% had experienced high levels of discrimination.
- 44.3% of MDR-TB patients who were employed, their levels of discrimination were high, whereas, for the 27.3% of unemployed patients, the levels of discrimination were high (17.3 per cent).
- Over half of the respondents (55.7% of respondents) were ineligible for employment according to the preceding table. This proportion of individuals who had a low level of discrimination, a moderate level of discrimination, and a high level of discrimination is roughly 18.7%, 10.4%, and 26.6% respectively.
- Approximately 56.1% of respondents were ineligible for any type of income as seen in the above table in this particular range, the amount of discrimination had a 17.4% rate of people with

low levels, a 10.4% rate of people with moderate levels, and a 26.6% rate of people with high levels.

- 75.4 per cent of respondents said that there was no family member support for patients with MDR-TB while 24.6 per cent reported having support.
- When it came to being isolated or discriminated against by family members, over six in ten respondents (61.6 per cent) reported being isolated, whereas over four in ten respondents (38.4 per cent) reported not being isolated or discriminated against by their family members. TB patients who are cared for by family members were found to consume food along with 47% of the time, but those who are cared for by others do so 53% of the time.

Level of Stigma Resistance

- It was found that older children and adolescents have greater levels of stigma resistance. Over the age of 18, 9.7% of the 24.6% of patients with MDR-TB were assessed to have low stigma resistance, while 3.8% and 11.1% were classified as having moderate levels of stigma resistance. Low-level stigma was felt by 25.3% of those aged 51 to 60, moderate-level stigma was experienced by 6.2%, and high-level stigma was experienced by 9% of the population in this age range.
- Majority (89.7%) were Hindus, with over 35% identifying as such and having higher levels of stigma resistance. It was found that Muslims made up approximately 5.5% of the population. In roughly 2.8% of the population, about two and a half per cent, people had significant levels of stigma resistance. And it was determined that Christians are only about 2.8% of the population some of those who showed high levels of stigma resistance, 0.7% of those reported being highly resilient.
- An estimated 33.2% of the population finished high school. Among those surveyed, 15.9% demonstrated poor stigma resistance, whereas 5.5% exhibited moderate stigma resistance. In a book that surveyed over 14,000 people, 11.8% exhibited a greater level of stigma resistance.

- Most of the patients (69.2%) were married. According to our research, 26.7% of respondents had poor stigma tolerance, 14.9% had light stigma tolerance, and 25.6% reported meeting greater stigma.
- The book findings show that MDR-TB patients who were employed (44.3 per cent) were more tolerant of discrimination than were unemployed patients (38.1 per cent) and people who were out of work (15.9 per cent).
- Among those who responded, more than half were found to be ineligible for work (55.7% of respondents). Low stigma resistance is seen in 22.1% of this category, moderate stigma resistance is in 10.4%, and high stigma resistance occurs in 23.2% of those in this category.
- It is 56.1% of the respondents were without income, indicating that they were ineligible for any money. 22.1% of patients reported resisting stigma, whilst 10.4% reported being moderately resistant to stigma. 23.5% of the participants reported experiencing strong levels of stigma resistance.
- One fourth (30.1%) of evidence of high-level stigma resistance was revealed in the research, which stated that 75.4% of respondents claimed that there was no family member assistance throughout the sickness of MDR-TB patients.
- When it came to isolation and discrimination by family members, over two-thirds of respondents (61.6 per cent) reported it, but only one-third (38.4 per cent) of respondents reported it wasn't true.

Level of ISDM

- The respondents' ages and ISDM levels varied. Patients aged 18 to 30 with MDR-TB comprised 24.6%, with 8.3% having low ISDM and 3.8% and 12.5% having moderate ISDM.
- The majority of respondents (91.7%) were Hindu, and among them (41.9%) had greater ISDM than Muslims and Christians. Muslims make up about 5% of the population. In the Muslimgroup, 3.1% showed "high levels of ISDM," while 1.4% had high levels in the Christian group.

- The overall percentage of patients with more than five family members was 4.5%, with low ISDM levels at 2.4%, moderate ISDM levels at 0.7%, and higher ISDM levels at 1.4%.
- According to the data, over half of the respondents (55.7%) were unemployed. In this location, 18.7% had low ISDM, 10.4% had moderate ISDM, and 26.6 had high ISDM.
- As stated previously, over half of the respondents (56.1%) were not eligible for any form of income.
- This group had low ISDM at 19%, moderate ISDM at 10.4%, and high ISDM at 26.6
- Threequarters (75.4%) of respondents reported no family assistance throughout MDR-TB patients' illness, while one-quarter (24.6%) reported no help at all.
- The majority of respondents (61.6%) reported being isolated and discriminated against by family members.

Discussion and Suggestion

The major findings of the book are presented in the first part of this chapter, which highlights the MDR patients' psychosocial well-being in terms of demographic and personal characteristics, socioeconomic status, TB treatment, family and institutional support, general health status, and self-stigma variables.

The second part of this chapter addresses the suggestions based on qualitative interviews with MDR-TB patients; a few important action points will promote and improve MDR-TB patients' psychosocial well-being in the country. The third section of the chapter concludes with future research directions. Serious psychosocial challenges are experienced by MDR-TB patients both due to disease and its treatment complexities.

A comparison of MDR-TB patients' overall health state, and self-stigma factors revealed major differences in their psychological well-being. It is important to educate the population on early symptoms and treatment options to reduce the number of new MDR-TB cases. For example, local government health officials and school teachers can encourage nutritional awareness among schoolchildren and community members. The MDR-TB patients who are registered for treatment and those who are sole breadwinners of their family can be provided with a monthly pension or monthly grant during the treatment period to improve their quality of life.

Lack of awareness is one of the major factors for poor health-seeking behaviours for TB therefore good community level awareness programme on TB is required to sensitize on early symptoms and treatment thereby preventing the number of new MDR-TB cases. People who live in unclean and poorly ventilated environments are more vulnerable to TB. Government housing projects such as the Pradhan Mantri Gramin Awas Yojana or the applicable State Government housing programme can be considered for the poor to enhance their living conditions and quality of life. The importance of TB patient and their family counselling should be strengthened by the health providers especially the counsellor to reduce psychological distress and self-stigma among the MDR-TB patients. In the National Tuberculosis Elimination Program, the appointment of a Medical Social Worker/Counsellor to coordinate MDR-TB treatment and provide psychological counselling has the potential to enhance adherence to treatment as well as the cure rate for MDR-TB patients.

Future Directions

- To begin with, we can examine the studies listed below; this research might lead to more detailed studies of the self-stigma among patients with multidrug-resistant tuberculosis (MDR-TB) in diverse locations, as well as identifying contributing factors.
- Such research in other countries and India could focus on MDR-TB patients' psychosocial well-being.
- Research that looks at adults is being done now; additional research including children who have contracted MDR-TB may ensue.
- To research, the well-being of MDR-TB patients in rural areas in future as this book only investigated the problem in urban areas. Additional investigation can be done for the respective patient populations, urban and rural.

- Stigma research in the book of self-stigma and how it manifests in gender, age MDR-TB patients is of particular interest.
- Research on psychological suffering in elements of MDR-TB may be done among patients who have that condition.
- People from different parts of the country could potentially be focusing on the socio-economic condition of MDR-TB patients in other cities and other parts of India.

Social Work Intervention

- Social worker will work as a bridge between TB patients and Health professionals; she/he will help the doctors in psychological intervention.
- Advocacy for psychosocial support and access to basic health services (Using wide publicity propaganda in social media about TB) functioning governance systems, into which psychosocial support needs to be mainstreamed, and the assurance of security in order to re-establish well-being and mitigate further psychosocial harm.
- Advertisement and educational references through Advocacy, Communication and Social Mobilization for TB.
- A smaller percentage of the population, with particularly stressful reactions, will require more focused and specialized support interventions with attention to the individual, family or group (e.g. psychosocial first aid by health workers, Medical Social workers).
- Good channels of communication should be established within the general hospital and with community services with regard to psychiatrics as well as physical health.
- Addressing psychological factors to ensure compliance is critical so the patients should be monitored for adverse drug reactions, which are common.
- Psychological, social and economic support interventions need to be included as a regular part of MDR-TB care.
- Depression during MDR-TB treatment needs particular attention. Health care professionals particularly Social worker

involved in management of MDR-TB patients should be properly skilled to execute proper mental health assessment tools, in particular at baseline, so that presence of depression can be identified on earlier basis.

- The social workers strive to eliminate discrimination, to reduced Psycho-Social issues and to promote the drug adherence by using the case work and group work social work intervention method among MDR-TB patients.
- Social workers engage in direct practice with patients in such roles as counsellor, enabler, case manager, and advocate.
- It is recommended to regularly monitor the mental health status of MDR-TB patients by skilled Medical Social Worker/ Counsellors using simple, validated and cost-effective tools which will result in adherence and cure rate in MDR-TB patients.
- The psychosocial and economic interventions conducted by Social worker will improve in both treatment adherence and cure rates among MDR-TB patients.

Conclusion

In addition, it has been found that the well-being of patients diagnosed with multidrug-resistant tuberculosis (MDR-TB) varies depending on age, gender, ethnicity, religion, social standing, personal attributes, and socioeconomic status. Poverty and illiteracy, when combined with several other factors, have an impact on a person's overall health, psychological well-being, and sense of personal shame. To achieve this there are many ways such as imparting basic education to all, providing employment opportunities, improving the health facilities, creating good health infrastructure facilities and involving various other stakeholders. Promotion of health facilities for the disease like TB and MDR-TB also would go a long way in addressing their health problems.

Social work is a problem-solving profession that uses a variety of methods, techniques, and approaches to assist individuals, groups, and communities in addressing problems. Around the world, policymakers, organizations, and governments are working hard to improve the health of TB and MDR-TB patients. This book could be very helpful for future social workers and other authorss who wish to perform further research on this topic, as it aims to improve MDR-TB patients' psychological well-being. To build on these preliminary findings and provide information on established psychosocial interventions that could be replicated in TB control programmes, large-scale multicenter investigations and randomised control trials are strongly recommended.

References

[1] Acha, J., Sweetland, A., Guerra, D., Chalco, K., Castillo, H., Palacios, E. (2007). Psychosocial support groups for patients with multidrug-resistant tuberculosis: Five years of experience. Global Public Health. *An International Journal for Research, Policy and Practice,* 2(4), 404–417.

[2] Anita, S. Mathew & Amol, M. Takalkar (2007). Living with Tuberculosis: The Myths and the Stigma from the Indian Perspective. *Clinical Infectious Disease,* 45(9), 1247.

[3] Balasubramanian, R., Garg, R., Santha, T., Gopi, P.G., Subramani, R., Chandrasekaran, V., Narayanan, P.R. (2004). Gender disparities in tuberculosis: report from a rural DOTS programme in South India. *International Journal Tuberculosis Lung Disease,* 8, 323–332.

[4] Baral, S.C., Karki, D.K., Newell, J.N. (2007). Causes of stigma and discrimination associated with tuberculosis in Nepal: A qualitative book. *BMC public health,* 7:211, 8.

[5] Baral, S.C., Aryal, Y., Bhattrai, R., King, R., Newell, J.N. (2014). The importance of providing counselling and financial support to patients receiving treatment for multi-drug resistant TB: Mixed method qualitative and pilot intervention studies. *BMC Public Health,* 14:46, 1–7.

[6] Basu, G., Chatterjee, C., Singh, R., Biswas, S. (2012). Prevalence of depression in tuberculosis patients: An experience from a DOTS clinic. *The Indian Journal of Research and Reports in Medical Sciences,* 2(4), 14-17.

[7] Booker, M.J. (1996). Compliance, coercion, and compassion: moral dimensions of the return of tuberculosis. *Journal of Medical Humanities,* 17(2), 91–102.

[8] Connolly, M. & Nunn, P. (1996). Women and tuberculosis. *World Health StatQ,* 49:115, 9.

[9] Fazlul Karim, A.M.R. Chowdhury, Akramul Islam and Mitchell G. Weiss. (2007). Stigma, Gender, and Their Impact on Patients with Tuberculosis in Rural Bangladesh. *Anthropology & Medicine,* 14(2), 139–151.

[10] Furin J. (2007). The clinical management of drug-resistant tuberculosis. *Current Opinion in Pulmonary Medicine,* 13(3), 212–7.

[11] Horter, Shona; Stringer, Beverley; Reynolds, Lucy; Shoaib, Muhammad; Kasozi Samuel; Casas, Esther C., *et al.* (2014). Home is

where the patient is: A qualitative analysis of a patient-centred model of care for multidrug-resistant tuberculosis. *BMC Health Services Research,* 14: 81, 1–8.

[12] Kaliakbarova, G., Pak, S., Zhaksylykova, N., Raimova, G., Temerbekova, B., Van den Hof, S. (2013). Psychosocial Support Improves Treatment Adherence Among MDR-TB Patients: Experience from East Kazakhstan. *The Open Infectious Diseases Journal*, 7, 60–64.

[13] Karl, Peltzer; Pamela, Naidoo; Gladys, Matseke; Julia, Louw; Gugu, Mchunu and Bomkazi, Tutshana (2012). Prevalence of psychological distress and associated factors in tuberculosis patients in public primary care clinics in South Africa. *BMC Psychiatry,* 12:89, 1–9.

[14] Long, N.H., Johansson, E., Diwan, V.K. and Winkvist, A. (2001). Fear and social isolation as consequences of tuberculosis in VietNam: A gender analysis. Health Policy, 58, 69–81.

[15] Morris, D.M., Quezada, L., Bhat, P., Moser, K., Smith, J., Perez, H., *et al.* (2013). Social, Economic, and Psychological Impacts of MDR-TB Treatment in Tijuana, Mexico: A Patient's Perspective. International Journal of Tuberculosis Lung Disease, 17 (7), 954–960.

[16] Nitesh, Kumar Singh; Pankaj, Kumar Gupta and Jai, Singh Yadav, Psychological Distress in Patients of Multi-Drug Resistant Tuberculosis International Journal of Health Sciences & Research (www.ijhsr.org) Vol. 9; Issue: 11; November 2019,

[17] Vega, P., Sweetland, A., Acha, J., Castillo, H., Guerra, D., Smith Fawzi, M.C. and Shin, S. (2004). Psychiatric issues in the management of patients with multidrug-resistant tuberculosis. *International Journal of Tuberculosis Lung Disease*, 8(6), 749–759.

[18] PekkaMartikainen, Mel Bartley, EeroLahema (2002). Psychosocial determinants of Health in Social Epidemiology. International Journal of Epidemiology, 31, 1091–1093.

[10] Rajeswari, R., Balasubramanian, R., Muniyandi, M., *et al.* (1999). Socio-economic impact of tuberculosis on patients and family in India. *International Journal of Tuberculosis and Lung Disease,* 3(10), 869–877.

[20] Rajeswari, R., Muniyandi, M., Balasubramanian, R. and Narayanan, P.R. (2005). Perceptions of tuberculosis patients about their physical, mental and social well-being: A field report from South India. *Social Science & Medicine*, 60, 1845-1853.

[21] Rameshchandra, M. Thakker and Gunjan, P. Upadhyay (2014). The psychosocial reaction of diagnosing tuberculosis – An experience of

tertiary care centre of rural Gujarat. International Journal of Medical Science and Public Health, 3, 12.

[22] Rubel, A.J. and Garro, L.C. (1992). Social and cultural factors in the successful control of Tuberculosis. Public Health Reports, 107(6), 626–636.

[23] Sudha, G., Nirupa, C., Rajasakthivel, *et al.* (2003). Factors influencing the care-seeking behaviour of chest symptomatic; a community-based book involving rural and urban population in Tamil Nadu, South India. Tropical Medicine & International Health, 8(4), 336–341.

[24] Drug-Resistant TB (MDR-TB) TB Guidelines, Centre for Disease Control and Prevention.

[25] Guidelines on Programmatic Management of Drug-Resistant TB (PMDT) in India-RNTCP2012.

[26] Guideline for PMDT in India 2017.

[27] NTEB—India TB Report- Central TB Division, New Delhi-2020.

[28] NTEP—Annual Report, Central TB Division, New Delhi-2020.

[29] National Strategic Plan for Tuberculosis Control 2012–2017.

[30] National Strategic Plan for Tuberculosis Elimination 2017–2025.

[31] Tuberculosis, WHO -Fact sheet October-2020

[32] WHO-Global Tuberculosis reports-1997–2020.

[33] WHO-Global Tuberculosis reports-2020.

Internet Sources

1. https://www.who.int/tb/public/
2. https://www.cdc.gov/tb/topic/drtb/default.htm
3. https://www.cdc.gov/tb/publications/factsheets/general/tb.htm, https://www.tbfacts.org/multi-drug-resistant-tb
4. https://en.wikipedia.org/wiki/Chennai
5. https://tbcindia.gov.in/showfile.php?lid=3322
6. https://apps.who.int/iris/bitstream/handle/10665/336069/97892400 13131-eng.pdf.
7. https://www.bing.com/search?q=Monoresistance+Tuberculosi&qs=n &form=QBRE&=1&pq=monoresistance+tuberculosi&sc=027&sk=& cvid=2A10457F2F30464F97292C75253D8087
8. https://www.thehealthsite.com/diseases-conditions/tuberculosis/tb-patients-should-get-covid-19-vaccine-as-early-as-possible-804164/
9. https://tbcindia.gov.in/WriteReadData/NSP%20Draft%2020.02.201 7%201.pdf

10. https://www.tbcindia.gov.in/WriteReadData/l892s/8337437943TOG-Chapter%204-Treatment%20of%20TB%20Part%201.pdf
11. http://www.who.int/tb/careproviders/ppm/IPAQT.pdf
12. https://tbcindia.gov.in/showfile.php?lid=3314
13. https://www.tbfacts.org/wp-content/uploads/2017/12/NSP-2012-2017.pdf
14. https://tbcindia.gov.in/showfile.php?lid=3319
15. http://www.who.int/tb/FDC_Factsheet.pdf
16. https://www.who.int/news-room/fact-sheets/detail/tuberculosis.
17. https://www.who.int/news-room/fact-sheets/detail/tuberculosis